My I

Irritable Bowel Sy

Michael Requim

Copyright Information

A Special Gift for Our Readers

Thank you for purchasing My Physician Guide to Irritable Bowel Syndrome. In addition to this incredible guide, you now have free access to our archive of bonus health, nutrition and fitness material. Simply visit the following link to claim your free bonus guides:

http://www.myphysician.com/bonus

Table of Contents

Introduction

Irritable Bowel Syndrome, or IBS, is a condition of the gastrointestinal tract characterized by severe abdominal pain, cramps, gas and bloating. Diarrhea and constipation are also common symptoms occurring in people with IBS. It is very prominent disease, affecting up to 20% of the world's population. It is the most common chronic health disorder in America, Canada, the United Kingdom, Australia and New Zealand, affecting more people than asthma, diabetes and depression combined.

IBS is considered to be a physical disorder despite the fact that two of the triggers are stress and anxiety. It is important to rule out other disorders to arrive at a conclusion of an IBS diagnosis. A number of other conditions, some of which are more serious, show the same initial symptoms as IBS. These include Crohn's disease and ulcerative colitis. Talking with your doctor and a gastrointestinal specialist can help pinpoint the problem.

There is no known cure for IBS, but there are ways to cope up with the problem and minimize the negative symptoms. Treatments include symptomatic medications, dietary adjustments, therapy to reduce stress, and changes in lifestyle. The most important thing to consider is that a patient has to be educated and dedicated to treatment in order for it to be successful. The relationship between the doctor and patient also plays as an important role in recovery as anything else.

The Digestive System

The digestive system consists of various organs working together to breakdown and absorb nutrients and expel waste and toxic substances from the body. The nutrients absorbed are used to build and nourish cells and to provide energy. The process begins in the mouth where food is ingested and ends at the anus where waste is expelled.

As food is chewed, it is mixed with saliva. Saliva is used to lubricate the material so it does not get stuck when travelling to the stomach. When this mixture is swallowed, the muscle movement begins and the food is pushed to the next levels of the digestive system. This movement of pushing the food is called peristalsis. The following are the steps involved in the digestion process.

After food is swallowed, it goes to the esophagus, or food pipe. This is the part of the tube that connects the mouth and the stomach.

At the entrance of the stomach there is a ring-like muscle which acts as a valve, opening to let food pass down but closing so it does not easily come back up.

The stomach mixes the food and liquid along with digestive juices to destroy bacteria and prepare the food for proper absorption. The food is mixed by the muscular contractions of the wall. The contents are then slowly released into the duodenum, the first section of the small intestine.

The small intestine absorbs the nutrients from the food via its walls that contain the blood stream flowing and these nutrients are transported throughout the body. From here, water and waste products are propelled to the large intestine. The large intestine compacts the waste materials and extracts any extra water. The collected products are sent on to the rectum where they rest until we discharge them through the anus. Two important muscles – the internal and external sphincter – keep the waste inside until we find a suitable time to pass them. The peristaltic contractions of the colon propel the waste out of the anus.

What Happens When this Process Goes Wrong?

When any one of these functions goes wrong, the whole process is disrupted. Researchers have found that while healthy people have between 68 contractions every 24 hours, persons suffering from Irritable Bowel Syndrome have about 25 contractions in the same period of time if they have diarrhea, and almost no contractions if they suffer from constipation. Problems related to IBS are not caused by inflammations or infections but from erratic or irregular muscle movements inside the body.

The contractions of the muscles of the colon are controlled by nerves and hormones. If the contractions of the colon do not match those of the sphincters and the pelvic muscles, the contents do not move in the proper way and cause the symptoms associated with IBS.

There are three main types of IBS and they are categorized according to their symptoms. In constipation predominant IBS, the rectum relaxes soon after a meal. The gastrocolic response is dull and the discomfort occurs at the lower rectal area. Diarrhea predominant IBS is characterized by an increase in rectal tone after a meal. The gastrocolic response is enhanced and there is a hypersensitivity to rectal distention. The third type is a combination of the two symptoms alternating in consecutive episodes.

Ruling out Serious Conditions

Irritable Bowel Syndrome is not a serious medical issue and does not permanently harm the intestines. However, the condition causes a great deal of discomfort and distress and the symptoms can appear to be similar to more serious conditions.

It is not possible for routine clinical tests to initially pinpoint the condition as IBS. Tests are performed more often to rule out other problems like inflammation, ulcers, cancer, parasites, celiac disease, fructose malabsorption, and endometriosis. Stool sample testing, blood tests, X-rays, sigmoidoscopies and colonoscopies are some tests that may be administered. Usually only after ruling out other diseases can one to the conclusion that it is IBS.

Risk Factors for IBS

Some risk factors have been identified to help alert a person to their vulnerability of contracting the condition:

- IBS most commonly affects teenagers or people in their twenties

- Hereditary factors: if someone in your family suffers from it you will be more likely to as well.

- If you suffer from recurrent infections of the digestive system

- Chronic stress or having psychological distress in the form of anxiety or depression. Note: stress management and behavior therapy has found to help relieve symptoms.

- People who suffer from other chronic pain syndromes like migraine headaches, chronic fatigue syndrome, fibromyalgia, and temporomandibular disorder.

- IBS has known to occur more often in women than men, and this prevalence has been attributed to the changing hormonal conditions in women.

- Eating quickly during high stress times or eating large meals has been found to affect an already hypersensitive colon.

- Some of the antibiotics, antidepressants and drugs containing sorbitol have been associated with IBS.

- Food poisoning can trigger the first onset of IBS symptoms. However, it may also be due to a sensitive colon being exposed to foods it has difficulty handling.

- Trapped gas which may cause bloating.

- Dietary issues such as food allergies and the amount of fiber consumed.

- Hypersensitivity of the nerve endings lining the colon tract.

- Malabsorption of bile acid.

- Inadequate physical activity.

- Chronic alcohol abuse.

- Abnormalities in the gastrointestinal secretions and/or peristalsis.

- Hormonal changes as in menstrual cycle.

- Excessive use of antibiotics.

- Substances like chocolate, milk products and caffeine may cause IBS if used excessively.

Symptoms of IBS

IBS symptoms vary depending on the type of IBS being expressed. The constipation predominant IBS is characterized by difficulty in passing stools while the diarrhea predominant IBS is known to have uncontrollable urgency to have a bowel movement. Someone with diarrhea predominant IBS will have three or more bowel movements in one day and someone with constipation predominant will only pass three or fewer bowel movements in one week.

There is also a feeling of incomplete evacuation. Mucus is present in the stool and one can experience bloating or flatulence. Sometimes, blood can be noticed in the stools. In persons with severe IBS, weight loss and severe pain is common. IBS sufferers have also been known to develop psychological problems, such as anxiety and depression, due to the painful experiences and inability to sometimes participate in social gatherings.

The abdominal pain in IBS is characterized by a few exclusive features. It is relieved by bowel movement, there is a change in the frequency of the bowel movement and also there is a change in the form, frequency and appearance of the stool. For the correct diagnosis of IBS, a history of symptoms must be present for at least 12 weeks, but not necessarily continuously.

These symptoms may come on gradually or may be triggered by an event resulting in sudden occurrence. Some events which have been known to cause IBS include bouts of food poisoning, a major surgery like a hysterectomy or cholecystectomy (removal of the gall bladder) or stressful periods of time such as after a breakup.

Once symptoms become present, flare ups may occur from certain triggers. These triggers may include large meals, medicines like antibiotics, drinks with caffeine, stress or emotional upsets etc. Some IBS sufferers may be sensitive to certain food items like wheat, rye, barley, chocolate, milk products or alcohol. The symptoms are known to be aggravated in women during or just before their menstrual cycle, suggesting the role of hormone levels plays an important part.

In patients with severe IBS, symptoms such as fever, vomiting, abdominal pain and cramping, poor appetite and fatigue are known to occur. The pain and cramping are not relieved by bowel movement, and may be so severe that it awakes the person from sleep.

Bacteria and the Immune System

The gastrointestinal tract is lined with different types of bacteria and varying concentrations depending on the organ and functions that needs to be served. The large intestine has over 700 species of bacteria that are helpful and useful. Some of them help in metabolizing undigested fiber into short chain fatty acids to be absorbed into the body, and some produce Vitamin K and biotin for absorption in the blood.

There are a group of bacteria that produce gas as a result of bacterial fermentation. This gas is a mixture of nitrogen and carbon dioxide and other gases. This gas is created as a byproduct of foods being broken down. Excess gas is expelled as flatulence.

Some bacteria trigger the immune system to produce cross reactive antibodies. These antibodies are also effective against related pathogens, and thus prevent infection. The American Journal of Gastroenterology found that IBS patients have a 72% increase in the immune system cells, and slightly lower immune system markers.

Sometimes, these bacteria can grow uncontrollably in the large intestine and may spread from the colon into the small intestine. Other times, one may have a deficient amount of the healthy bacteria. This may cause excess gas, abdominal bloating, distension, diarrhea and abdominal pain. Routinely taking probiotics can help regulate the amount of "good" bacteria in the intestines.

IBS and Other Similar Conditions

Irritable bowel syndrome is diagnosed only after excluding the presence of other conditions that have similar symptoms. The diagnosis of IBS is possible if the following is done:

- Carefully going through the history and physical examination

- Inflammation needs to be checked

- Celiac disease can be ruled out from a serological testing

- Stool culture for infection or growth may be checked

- Family history of inflammatory bowel disease or colon cancer has to be checked

- Lactose intolerance testing to rule out the specific intolerance

- Presence of the symptoms for more than 12 weeks, not essentially consecutively

The conditions that have similar symptoms include:

- Inflammatory bowel disease

- Abuse of antacids or laxatives

- Lactose intolerance

- Parasitic infestation

- Diverticulitis

- Addison's disease

- Gallstones

- Gastro esophageal reflux disease

- Malabsorption syndrome such as celiac disease or long term pancreatitis

Certain laboratory test procedures and radiographic studies would reveal the presence of pathological or physical abnormalities that would exclude irritable bowel syndrome. For example, gastrointestinal bleeding has to be ruled out with a hematocrit test, and microbiological tests on stool samples check for ova and parasites. Breath tests rule out bacterial overgrowth, lactose/fructose intolerance, and abnormalities of the thyroid. Imaging studies like an upper GI barium study would rule out tumors, inflammation, obstructions, and Crohn's disease. An ultrasonography test of the gall bladder can be performed if persistent indigestion and pain is present. An abdominal CT scan could rule out tumors, obstruction and pancreatic disease.

An endoscopy is generally suggested for patients with irritable bowel syndrome as a flexible sigmoidoscopy, to determine inflammation or distal obstruction. Endoscopy of the whole GI tract with possible biopsy is indicated for a patient with persistent dyspepsia or any symptoms that suggest malabsorption. A colonoscopy is necessary for patients with warning signs such as bleeding, anemia, chronic diarrhea, and history of colon polyps or cancer.

Since IBS is characteristically diagnosed as an irritation in the bowels in the absence of any pathological or physical abnormalities, it is sometimes considered to be psychosomatic or functional disorder.

IBS and Candida

Candida is a form of yeast or fungus that can grow uncontrollably in the digestive system. This can also spread and proliferate throughout the body by the bloodstream, resulting in a condition known as Candidiasis. The symptoms of Candidiasis and irritable bowel syndrome have been found to be similar except for yeast infections, rectal itching and thrush (an infection of the mouth), which occurs in the former condition.

Candida is nurtured by a diet high in sugar content as the yeast feeds on ingested sugar. The growth of yeast may also be facilitated when the 'good' bacteria that suppresses its growth is destroyed by the abuse of antibiotics. Also, a repressed immune system paves the way for uncontrolled fungal growth in the digestive tract. Using birth control pills and excessively engaging in processed foods have also known to cause candidiasis.

The mucosal lining of the gastrointestinal tract can get porous because of the invasion of this fungus. This results in the improper absorption of food particles in the bloodstream causing toxic and allergic reactions. The condition is commonly known as "leaky gut".

The yeast can thus spread out to various organs in the body and cause inflammations and conditions like fungal toenails, thrush, sinusitis and others. The fungus is very adaptable to all kinds of environment and spreads easily.

Although, IBS can be contracted without having candidiasis, many believe that candidiasis may trigger IBS. Elimination of the yeast through diet, medication and probiotics will no doubt help prevent the onset and flare ups of IBS.

Food and IBS

Foods to Avoid

One of the many triggers of IBS is food. However, there is no certain specific list of food that one has to avoid. The trigger foods need to be identified for each individual and be avoided.

Certain foods and eating practices that aggravate the symptoms of IBS include natural honey, refined sugar or artificial sweeteners, dairy products, fried foods, red meat, egg yolks, and products containing caffeine. Some foods cause gas and bloating that, in turn, lead to the aggravation of IBS symptoms are banana, raisins, onion, beans, garlic, and bagels.

Fat seems to be the widely accepted culprit to trigger irritable bowel syndrome. It is though that when fat enters the stomach, it sets off the gastrocolic reflex, which causes contractions of the colon to propel contents further. The muscle spasms triggered by fats result in fast contractions and the contents are rushed through the colon without enough time to absorb water. If the condition is IBS constipation predominant, fecal matter is not able to move but the contractions occur and result in excessive pain.

Fiber is important to anyone with IBS. Soluble fiber is found in foods considered starchy such as grains and cereals. A supplement is also a good source of fiber if you cannot get enough naturally. Soluble fiber soothes and regulates the digestive tract, controls the colon contractions and helps regulate bowel movements. Fiber is the primary cause of stool consistency – too much and material will easily pass through you and result in diarrhea. Too little fiber and you will have constipation. Insoluble fiber, on the other hand, is a stimulant of the GI tract and can irritate the bowel and is best had in combination with the foods that contain soluble fiber. It is not healthy to totally eliminate the insoluble fiber from the diet.

Keeping a food log will alert you to the foods that cause you problems. Most IBS sufferers have to avoid or eliminate certain types of food that trigger symptoms. Record the symptoms, duration, intensity of effects and what you ate prior to symptoms in your log. Show this log to your doctor to discover which foods may be causing you discomfort.

Foods You Need and Nutrition Tips

Foods that contain soluble fiber should be eaten first, on an empty stomach, and also must form a large part of every meal.

Eat smaller meals more frequently throughout the day instead of 3 large meals at breakfast, lunch and dinner.

The fat intake should be kept to a minimum. Foods high in fats (fried foods) must be avoided.

Try substituting low fat vegetarian versions of meat products, bread spreads can be fruit purees instead of butter, cheese or margarine, veggie broth instead of oil in sauces and herbs and spices can be added to enhance flavors to be enjoyed instead of oils and fats.

Instead of eating raw vegetables, which are rich in insoluble fiber, eat them as soups, purees or simply boiled. This breaks up the insoluble fiber and makes them more acceptable in the GI tract.

Drink at least eight 8oz cups of water each day. Some of this water can be substituted for milk and juice too. Caffeinated beverages like coffee are diuretics which will make you urinate more and will actually lower the amount of water in your body. Remaining well hydrated will help you feel better and will promote good digestion.

Dining Tips if you suffer from IBS

It is important to stay calm and stress free if you are planning to eat out or eat a meal with some unhealthy foods. Use various relaxation methods like meditation, deep breathing, and muscle relaxation techniques. You don't want your anxiety to compound the effects of the food to potentially trigger more powerful symptoms.

Just in case, know the location of the bathroom in the restaurant before you settle in for your meal. Also have transportation available in case you need to leave in an emergency. It may sound silly, but visualize the evening before it begins. Imagine yourself calmly eating dinner without any IBS symptoms. This will help you reduce stress for the evening and could help prevent a future attack.

Some people believe that depriving themselves of food before a meal can calm the digestive system. This is not necessarily true. Digestive contractions are a continuous process and occur even when food is not being digested. Small frequent meals containing soluble fiber can calm down the digestive system beforehand and also regulate your hunger levels so you won't binge when the big meal comes. Because fiber gives a feeling of fullness it is goods for those who wish to lose weight, control cholesterol and regulate blood sugar levels.

Select only those kinds of foods that do not upset your GI tract. If you politely explain to the waiter that you have a digestive disorder and you need to know the ingredients of a meal and how it is prepared, they will usually be very accommodating. If a particular meal is fried, ask for it grilled instead. If it contains large amounts of fat ask to have it lean.

If you have an emergency, kindly excuse yourself from the table. If you must leave abruptly you can explain to your party when you return so they do not think you were being rude. Not excusing yourself could set you up for an even bigger embarrassment.

More Facts on Fiber

Insoluble fiber speeds up the movements of the contents of the GI tract and facilitates regularity of defecation. It also adds bulk to the stool and helps rid of constipation.

Recommendations from the United States National Academy of Sciences, Institute of Medicine, say that an average adult must consume 2035 grams of dietary fiber per day. Soluble fiber can be found in legumes, oats, rye, barley, some fruits and juices, certain vegetables such as broccoli and carrots, root tubers and root vegetables and psyllium seed husk. Insoluble fiber can be found in whole grain foods, wheat and corn bran, nuts and seeds, flax seed, vegetables such as green beans and cauliflower, fruits such as avocado and bananas, skins of some fruits such as tomatoes, etc.

Irritable bowel syndrome, generally being the problem with movement of the contents, can be treated by the presence of dietary fiber, both soluble and insoluble. Soluble fiber absorbs water to form a gel and this prevents diarrhea. It also helps keep the GI tract muscles stretched gently around a full colon. It also enables the contents of the bowels to move smoothly upon being flushed and prevents violent and irregular spasms of the colon.

Insoluble fiber must never be eaten on an empty stomach or you will have gastrointestinal discomfort. One cannot completely avoid insoluble fiber as it can lead to other serious problems, so combine sources with other foods. Eating them with a larger serving of soluble fiber foods is the best way to reduce the bad effects of insoluble fiber.

Probiotics and Irritable Bowel Syndrome

"Pro" means "for" and "bios" means "life", thus, probiotic means "for life". This is a term that has been used to describe nutritional supplements that contain live bacteria in recommended dosages. Acidophilus is one such friendly bacteria that can boost intestinal flora and stabilize the intestines and provide relief from irritable bowel syndrome. Bifido bacterium and lactobacillus are two such well known bacteria that help in soothing the intestinal muscles. Probiotics are beneficial for a number of reasons:

- Prevent the growth of harmful fungus and yeast in the GI tract.

- Help keep the stool soft, well formed and facilitates peristalsis.

- Help prevent GI tract infections.

- Produce vitamins B and K and Lactase (enzyme that digests milk and dairy products).

- Remove gas and excess waste.

- Balance sex hormones and improves fertility.

- Control growth of pathogenic bacteria and viruses.

- Suppress toxins and produces antibodies and anti-carcinogens.

- Prevent cholesterol from entering the blood stream and lower blood pressure.

- Bring a balance to the immune system

- Reduce dental cavities.

- Aid in weight loss.

- Strengthen bones and keep them healthy.

- Help control acne.

There are various foods that are natural sources of probiotics. These include soft cheeses, miso soups, yogurts, sauerkraut, tempeh or fermented soy, and buttermilk. Probiotic supplements are also available in the market mostly in the form of capsules, tablets, liquids, and powders.

How to Stock an IBS-Friendly Kitchen

There are some IBS friendly foods that should be stocked in a kitchen. Brown rice, almond, coconut, potato flours, beans, peas, carrots, grains like buckwheat, millet, quinoa and amaranth are good for the IBS prone GI tract. They have enough soluble fiber to soothe the muscles of the intestines. Intestine friendly snacks include rice cakes, baked organic corn chips, baked potato chips, soaked nuts like cashew, almonds, pecans and macadamia nuts, and fruits like applesauce and bananas.

Drinks are the answers for untimely hunger pangs, and homemade smoothies and broths of chicken, vegetable and beef can be used. Breakfast cereals that can be used safely by IBS sufferers include oats and oatmeal, rice puffs, millet puffs and kamut puffs. Lunch items can include gluten and dairy free frozen meals. Safe sources of proteins include lean ground beef and turkey, chicken breasts, canned salmon, tofu and fish.

Dietary Supplements for IBS

Aloe Vera: Aloe vera is known to contain about 75 nutrients including vitamins, minerals, amino acids and enzymes that are essential for keeping good health overall. It also has anti-inflammatory attributes which are very effective in calming the intestinal spasms and sudden contractions of the intestines.

Chamomile: It is a perennial herb that has been extensively used throughout history. It is well known for being a mild sedative and has antispasmodic properties. This combination makes it ideal for soothing the muscles of the intestine, and has been proven to reduce irritation and cramping in animals. It is consumed as tea, a capsule or a tincture. The dosage depends on the form in which it is taken as recommended by a qualified physician or health care professional.

Evening Primrose Oil: this oil is extracted from the seeds, roots, leaves and flowers of the evening primrose. It is known to aid in digestion and reduce inflammation in the digestive tract. Three doses of

10002000 mg should be taken every day with food. However, the oil is known to interfere with medications used to treat epilepsy.

Peppermint: History speaks volumes about use of peppermint tea for treating general digestive disorders and reduction of gas in the intestines. The enteric coated peppermint oil capsules are effective in relieving pain, distension and stool frequency. It is consumed as capsules or as tea.

Psyllium: It is known to produce bulky soluble fiber that helps smooth bowel movements. However, it has to be introduced into the diet very gradually. Ideally, a few teaspoons along the normal intake of eight glasses of water a day can relieve diarrhea and constipation.

Calcium and Magnesium: These two minerals play an important role in regulating muscle function and provide the mechanism for muscle contraction and relaxation. While calcium has a constipating effect, magnesium works as a laxative. Usually a ratio of calcium to magnesium as 2:1 is ideal to keep this system working smoothly.

Digestive enzymes: They are usually taken before a meal, especially if the fat content of the meal is more than usual. Enzymes are available for foods that are known to produce gas like beans, lentils and a few vegetables.

Recipes for IBS Sufferers

Banana smoothie with egg whites: Combine 1 firm ripe banana, 1 egg white, ¼ rice milk or vanilla soy and 2 tablespoons of carob powder in a blender and puree until smooth. Pour in a glass and serve. Makes a great fast and easy breakfast that is rich in soluble fiber and low in fat.

Cream of Tomato soup with Basil meatballs: This recipe can be made using a lot of vegetables, lean turkey, egg white and tofu. Cook onion, garlic and water over low heat. When it turns tender, add bell peppers also. Stir in crushed tomatoes, tomato puree, orange zest, orange juice and water and bring to boil. Cook uncovered in low heat to blend the flavors. Process half of the basil leaves and pumpkin seeds until finely chopped. Mix in turkey, egg white, parmesan, pumpkin seed oil and salt and shape into walnut size meatballs. Drop this into the simmering soup and cook. Add pureed tofu to the soup to make it thick and creamy.

Butternut Brown rice Pilaf: Combine one and a half diced butternut squashes, 1 cup brown rice, 1 cup chicken broth, ¼ cup water and ¾ tablespoon curry powder and bring to boil over high heat. Now, cover and cook in a simmered flame for about 25 minutes till it is done. Stir in ¼ pound green beans and cook over low heat for five minutes, when the rice is just tender. Mix in the chopped basil leaves.

Potatoes roasted with garlic: Peel and quarter the potatoes and place them in a large nonstick skillet. Add cold water up to ¾ heights of the potatoes. Add 1 tablespoon olive oil, minced garlic cloves and 1 teaspoon of garlic salt and bring to boil. Reduce to medium heat and cook till water evaporates completely, stirring occasionally to cook the potatoes. Increase the heat and stir fry the potatoes till they are crispy. They taste best if eaten immediately.

Green tea: A simple ginger tea made by squeezing a fresh ginger and adding it to hot water and honey gives you a fabulous tea and also stimulates digestion, cleanses bowels and kidney along with its other benefits. Peppermint green tea can be made by placing ½ cup fresh mint leaves, 2 tablespoon sugar and 2 cups boiling water in a teapot and stir to dissolve sugar. Steep for 3 minutes and add ½ teaspoon of tea powder and let steep for 1 minute. Serve hot or chilled. Other ingredients used for making herbal teas are chamomile, orange, roses, jasmine, fennel, hibiscus, rosemary, vetiver, nettles, citrus blossoms, thyme licorice and others. However, one needs to identify the effect of the ingredient used on their intestines.

Baked root vegetables: Bake root vegetables like carrots, beets, turnips, parsnips, rutabagas, potatoes etc that are peeled and cut into 1 inch pieces. Pour in a tablespoon of olive oil and salt and toss the vegetables. Roast the mixture for about 30 minutes, stirring twice in between and add garlic cloves. Continue roasting for another 15 minutes, stirring once, till the vegetables are tender and browned. Seasoning can be done with chopped herbs like basil or mint. This can be had as a salad for dinner or a midevening snack.

<u>Grilled eggplant</u> Grill or broil a medium sized eggplant after pricking at several places with a fork to prevent bursting. The eggplant must be charred all over and very soft. After it cools down, discard the skin and blend the pulp with 1 cup cooked chickpeas, 1 large garlic clove, 2 tablespoons well stirred tahini, ¼ teaspoon salt and ¼ cup fresh lemon juice until you get a smooth puree. Transfer to serving bowl and sprinkle with parsley. This can be had with fresh pita bread.

The Power of Shakes and Smoothies

When you are grounded at home due to the troublesome irritable bowel syndrome, you have to resort to home cooked meals too. That is when the shakes, smoothies, juices and beverages come to aid, especially when you need something done in a short amount of time. These shakes and smoothies often involve more than one fruit and are very nutritious apart from being filling. Smoothies provide healthy carbohydrates, abundant vitamins, minerals, phytochemicals and also chlorophyll. The soluble fiber being the essential bulk of fruits and whey can help regulate the bowel movements and you will be free to go out sooner than you think.

These drinks can be made right at your home and you do not have to resort to liquid food supplements in the market that are full of unwanted chemicals like preservatives, additives and colors.

The fruits and vegetables have to be washed, cut, peeled and the core extracted before putting them into the blender. Generally, all the ingredients of the recipe are to be blended together unless indicated otherwise. Garnish them with lemon juice, parsley, coriander, cinnamon etc to enhance the taste as well as nutrient value.

The ingredients used in a juice can be a single fruit or a combination of two or more fruits to make a "mocktail." Fruits most commonly used in making juices are watermelon, orange, pineapple, berries, lemon, lime and grapefruits. Smoothies are generally made of fruits like bananas, apples, kiwi fruit, mango, coconut, papaya and berries like blueberry, strawberry and raspberry. A green smoothie is made of 40% dark green leafy vegetables and 60% fruits. Vegetables like cucumber, red cabbage, celery, and spinach make a smoothie more nutritious and contain less sugar.

Various ingredients used to thicken fruits and vegetable smoothies include nonfat frozen yogurt, ice, coffee, soymilk in various flavors, reduced fat coconut milk and many others. Some fruits like bananas, apples and mangoes are themselves thick in the form of a pulp. Adding yogurt increases the nutrient value as well as provides the much needed probiotic bacteria.

Stress and Irritable Bowel Syndrome

The stress response, as such, is a complicated process. It involves our nervous system and the endocrine system, which in turn bring about changes in the functioning of a variety of body processes. When the body reacts to a stressful situation, the hormone called cortisol is released. The autonomic nervous system triggers the release of adrenaline and noradrenaline that cause cardiovascular, muscular and digestive system changes. Both these pathways directly affect the network of nerves found in the bowels. Thus the cycle of stress and IBS is established in the body.

The intestinal contractions or spasms occur either too fast or too slow. If a meal is eaten while feeling stressed, the spasms are triggered, and the symptoms of diarrhea or constipation manifest. Exposure to a stressful situation also leads to gas formation, which in turn leads to bloating, cramping and pain. In severe cases, the intestines may get entangled and bleeding may occur.

A study by Drossman and his colleagues revealed that about 70% of people without IBS symptoms reported that they suffered from changes in bowel function as a reaction to stressful situations and some experienced abdominal pain and discomfort under stress conditions. However, it has been found that the people suffering from IBS are more prone to the gut reactions under stress than the others. IBS sufferers also tend to have a lower threshold for coping with stressful situations and are more likely to react to negative events.

De-stress Your Self and Get Relief

Sleep is an important factor in relaxation and rejuvenation. It is the most relaxed state of the body and the time when most of the complicated repairs take place. At least 8 hours of sleep every day, on a regular schedule, is required for the body to rest and repair itself.

Yoga is proven to be highly effective in handling stress. Yoga is a system of exercises that are physical as well as mental, and incorporates breathing patterns, exercises to improve flexibility of the body and meditation. This system aims to bring in a balance between the mind and the body and is known to provide a number of significant health benefits and improve longevity. Yoga is known to be beneficial to endocrinal disorders also and the consequences of stress related hormones and chemicals are easily overcome. Different yoga postures help in relieving the various symptoms of IBS like abdominal pain, spasms, gas formation, diarrhea and constipation, and other digestive disorders also.

Certain postures or yoga have also found to be helpful to relieve bloating:

Kneel on both knees and sit on your heels. Lean forward to rest your chest on your thighs. Place forehead on the floor and arms alongside the body, palms up and fingers pointing towards your feet. Breathe deeply through the nose for 5 minutes.

The cobra posture involves lying down on your stomach and lifting the upper body rising up on your hands. Take a deep breath and hold for eight seconds. Bring the upper body back to the floor breathing slowly along eight counts. After three sets, stand up and pat your stomach gently until you burp enough to release the gas trapped.

The "Rag Doll" posture involves standing erect and raising both hands high above head while breathing deeply. Bend down and try to touch the ground to the maximum possible extent, keeping your legs and knees straight. Allow your body to relax. Now, slowly twist your waist to move the body to the right side. Exhale in this position and inhale as you come back to center. Repeat on the left side without rising up. After three sets, stand up and pat your stomach until you burp.

Acupuncture, a form of traditional Chinese medicine, involves insertion of needles at target points. This is done by a trained and qualified practitioner using sterile needles and it is known to be safe and effective. Scientists speculate that acupuncture affects the nervous system by stimulating release of endorphins and also altering the blood circulation within the brain to increase the flow to the thalamus.

Heat therapy is used as a relaxant and is beneficial to IBS sufferers to overcome abdominal pains and cramps. Jacuzzis, steam baths or saunas have been found to help relieve the contractions of the colon and give quick relief. Heating pads, hot water bottles and long hot baths are other ways. Therapeutic massage manipulates the muscles and other soft tissues, and can help stimulate the peristalsis to reduce symptoms. However, massage should not be used during an acute episode of IBS or any other similar condition.

The IBS Emergency Kit

One thing to be remembered is that one must not allow the IBS to take over their life. Always be prepared for any kind of emergency. Some may consider wearing incontinence briefs in case you are prone to accidents. An IBS emergency kit should be on hand for a clean up after an accident. The kit should include a change of clothing and underwear, baby wipes (with perfume if required), a Ziploc bag for soiled underwear, deodorant spray and ant diarrhea medicine.

Exercise and IBS

While sleep plays an important role, active exercises also help in reducing stress levels. Regular exercise not only aids in digestion, but it also plays an important role in boosting the immune system, strengthening the muscles, increasing flexibility and promoting circulatory system health. Regular physical activity will help you sleep faster and deeper, which in itself is one of the best stress relievers.

Exercising at home or at the gym enables one to spend time on their own or socialize with others. Regular exercise reduces muscular pains, regulates blood circulation and digestion, decreases body fat, improves appetite for healthy foods, and boosts your energy levels. There are fun ways to exercise too. Ballroom dancing, hiking and trekking, games like tennis, football, etc, and other such physical activity incorporated into the daily schedule can be as good as working out at the gym.

Brisk walking, jogging, or swimming is recommended on a regular basis for 30 minutes, at least 4 days a week. The exercise should be such that your breathing rate and heart rate must rise significantly, about 60% above your normal rate. You should still be able to hold a conversation without tiring. Hiring a personal trainer or working out at the gym are the ways one can be motivated to continue the exercise programs for a longer time.

When to See a Specialist

You should regularly talk to your doctor about your IBS but you may need to see a specialist. Seeing a specialist is required if the symptoms persist for at least 12 months and/or if your condition worsens.

Certain characteristics of the stool are also indicative of irritable bowel syndrome. Abnormal stool frequency such as more than three bowel movements per day or less than three bowel movements in a week is one such indicator. The abnormal stool form is defined as the stool being lumpy and hard or loose and watery.

Abnormal defecation, characterized by straining or urgency or feeling of incomplete evacuation is usually the symptoms of constipation or diarrhea. Passage of mucus in the stool or feeling of abdominal distension and bloating may occur. The specialist may order tests like a colonoscopy, barium enema, sigmoidoscopy or upper GI series, to fully understand your situation.

Pharmaceutical Help

The drugs used for managing the symptoms of IBS are usually those dealing with neurotransmitters found in the intestinal system preventing symptoms of constipation or diarrhea, antispasmodics, antidepressants and analgesics. The medications given will depend on whether the IBS is diarrhea predominant or constipation predominant.

In the case of diarrhea predominant IBS, the treatment must aim to reduce the muscle contractions. The neurotransmitters within the intestines regulate the muscle contractions, mucus secretion and fluid absorption and other processes involved in digestion. The symptoms of diarrhea predominant IBS are managed by drugs such as Lotronex, Zofran, Kytril and Remeron, which target the specific receptor sites for certain neurotransmitters found in the gut. While Zofran and Kytril work to reduce nausea and vomiting associated with cancer treatment, the drug Remeron is an antidepressant. The drug Lotronex has been found to be responsible for serious side effects and is used only for women with severely unmanageable diarrhea predominant IBS and as a last resort.

Antispasmodic drugs like Bentyl (dicyclomine), Levbid & Levsin (hyoscyamine), Donnatol (belladonna/phenobarbital) and Buscopan (butylscopolamine) target the neurotransmitter acetylcholine and eventually help in reducing the contractions of the muscles in the intestines, as well as secretion of mucus. However, they are known to have side effects like dry mouth and dry eyes, urinary retention, tachycardia, drowsiness and mild constipation. Diarrheal urgency and incontinence can be managed by Imodium, Kaopectate and Maalox (all Loperamide), Pepto Bismol (bismuth subsalicylate), but they may also cause side effects like drowsiness, and constipation.

The symptoms of constipation-predominant IBS are relieved by drugs like Amitiza, Zelnorm and Lactulose. Amitiza increases the amount of fluids in the intestines by activating the proteins involved in transporting chloride. It is contraindicated in cases of bowel obstruction, severe diarrhea or pregnancy or if you are breastfeeding. Lactulose, the osmotic laxative, is a manufactured sugar that is broken down by bacteria in the intestines and pulls in more water in the colon and softens the stool. The softness of the stools and higher volume facilitates the motility of the colon, relieving constipation. Lactulose is contraindicated if the patient is scheduled for surgery, is diabetic, pregnant or is breastfeeding. Zelnorm is generally used to treat chronic idiopathic constipation and works by increasing the amount of the neurotransmitter serotonin in the nervous system of the gut. However, this is known to cause very serious side effects.

Over-the-counter drugs such as peppermint oil, herbs, probiotics and slippery elm help in overall digestion. Constipation can be addressed with magnesium, stool softeners, flaxseed, triphala and diarrhea symptoms can be handled with calcium and Imodium.

An IBS Diary

Since symptoms recur and are triggered by various conditions, IBS sufferers should keep a log. Write down these headings next to columns with a blank space next to each line. Record the time next to each entry for:

- Food eaten, and quantity.

- Mental work/stress levels/emotional factors

- Symptoms that have occurred time, severity (can be rated on a scale of 1 to 10)

- Any liquid beverages and drinks time, quantity, sugar content

- Number of glasses of water taken

- Medications and supplements taken

- Activities done and energy levels

Remember to write down everything that you eat and be honest about it. Include all drinks like coffee, tea, alcohol, soft drinks and others. This will help you identify triggers. Sometimes it may not be the individual foods that cause the trouble, but the ingredients used in the recipe, like excess fat or presence of gluten. Also, consider the correlation between your stress levels and presentation of symptoms.

Once the possible problematic triggers are identified, eliminate them completely for a period of time and see if the symptoms persist. Although the process is a long one and may take more than a month, it will surely help in the long term. Remember to take the diary to your doctor on your next visit. This will give him more insight into your problems and he will be able to better customize treatment.

Finding Support

Since you may require help from family and friends it is best to be open and explain your condition thoroughly. Be as precise as possible and let them know how it affects you, your outings, work and dating. This will help them know that IBS is a real illness that could impact not only your life but theirs as well. Sometimes, your IBS can cause your family or friends late for an event, a presentation or meeting. If they know about this condition, they can accommodate the unwarranted changes more easily.

Certain things for the friends, family, coworkers and superiors to know are:

- that you have a very real, chronic illness, diagnosed by a medical practitioner.

- that your symptoms may flare up at odd times, causing adjustments to your schedules.

- that you have no control over it

- that your doctor has understood and diagnosed the condition.

- that you have proof and reports and educational materials that is indicative of a physical condition.

- that you are working to address the problem but may need help

- that you will put in your best efforts to minimize the need for help and that their help is much appreciated.

The Internet: A Great Source of Help

Most IBS sufferers feel embarrassed to talk openly about their condition. For this reason, support groups can be a good way to get help and advice. IBS does not have to feel isolating if you have someone to help you through it. Various sources of information can be found online:

- Blogs that provide information and a place to comment

- Forums to interact with people with IBS and share experiences

- Articles about IBS mention and breakthroughs

- Interesting IBS-friendly recipes that have been tried and tested by the patients themselves.

- Downloadable food dairies

- A place to research treatments

The following are a list of support groups and forums to vent or find help from other IBS sufferers:

www.ibsgroup.org www.helpforibs.com
www.ibspage.com www.ibstales.com
www.ibssupport.ning.com www.ibshelp-
online.com/ibsforum.html
www.facebook.com/ibsgroup
www.revolutionhealth.com/ibsselfhelpandsupport-
group www.guttrust.org www.forums.about.com/ab-
ibs/

Conclusion

Irritable bowel syndrome does cause a lot of distress if you have the condition but it does not have to control your live. Many changes must occur and with perseverance and strength you can stay in control. You must identify the trigger foods and eliminate them from diet, listen to all doctor advice, follow medications, take the required supplements and probiotics, exercise often and sleep well. Managing the syndrome won't be easy and major lifestyle changes will need to occur but have hope because it is still possible to have a long, happy and fulfilling life with IBS.

The Healthy Eating Power Guide

One of the most critical ways you can significantly improve your health is through a proper diet. Whether faced with a serious medical condition or not, eating the right foods can make a major difference in how your body reacts to problems. A proper diet can improve the body's ability to ward off invading bacteria, improve immune system functioning, and help the body to avoid future complications. For this reason we have included this Healthy Eating Power Guide to provide you with dieting tips and nutrition strategies to help you reach your health goals. Note that some medical conditions require a special diet as prescribed by a physician or nutritionist and you should consult with your health practitioner to make sure your diet will work for you.

Assessing your Nutritional Profile

Most people are anxious to improve their diets, but in today's hectic, fast food oriented world, eating healthy can be quite a challenge. Our goal with this guide is to help you make smart food choices while still enjoying your life and your family.

Making your everyday diet a healthier one is one of the best things you can do to improve the way you look, and the way you feel, and possibly even how long you live. So why not get started today with a healthier eating lifestyle?

Everyone wants to eat a healthier diet, but it can sometimes be difficult to know if your diet is healthy enough. There are a number of factors that go into creating a healthy diet, and it is important to evaluate the current state of your diet before embarking on a plan for healthier eating.

There are several questions you should ask yourself when evaluating the healthiness (or lack thereof) of your current eating plan. These questions include:

Do I eat a wide variety of foods?

Variety is one of the most important hallmarks of a healthy diet, since no one food contains all the nutrients needed by the human body. It is important to eat foods from all the major food groups, including grains and breads, fruits and vegetables, milk and dairy products, meats, beans and nuts. If you find yourself avoiding some food groups, such as vegetables for instance, it may be time to look for a healthier diet.

Do I recognize the importance of cereals, breads and other grain products?

Eating a wide variety of grain based products is important to a healthy diet. Grains and cereals contain a large number of important nutrients, including high levels of dietary fiber. They also contain rich sources of starch, which provide our main sources of energy.

It is important to choose whole grain products as often as possible, since whole grain products like wheat bread contain more nutrients than more refined white bread and similar products. When eating cereal, it is a good idea to choose whole grain varieties, or those that are enriched with vitamins and minerals.

Do I eat lots of fruits and vegetables?

Many people do not eat sufficient servings of fruits and vegetables every day. Most experts recommend eating between 5 and 9 servings of fruits and vegetables every day, roughly equivalent to 2 cups of fruit and 2 ½ cups of vegetables.

When shopping for vegetables and fruits, it is important to choose a good variety of dark green, dark red, orange and yellow varieties. That is because different colored fruits and vegetables contain a variety of different nutrients, including vitamin C, vitamin A and beta carotene.

Do I eat a good breakfast every morning?

Breakfast, or the absence of it, is often a good indicator of the state of your diet. If you rush out of the house every morning and grab a donut at the local convenience store, chances are your diet can use some work. A healthy breakfast provides a foundation for the rest of the day, helps you avoid cravings and provides much needed nutrition.

Do I choose low fat foods over higher fat alternatives?

This is also an important question to ask yourself. Low fat alternatives are available for a variety of products, including milk, cheese, meats and more.

One part of following a healthy, low fat diet is avoiding prepared foods whenever possible, since prepared foods tend to have higher amounts of fat and sodium than fresh foods.

It is also important to control the amount of fat that is added at the table. Adding things like butter, sour cream and heavy sauces is a sure way to ruin an otherwise healthy meal. Even healthy foods like salads can be sabotaged by the addition of high fat salad dressings. Try using lower fat alternatives like flavored vinegars instead.

Do I drink plenty of water?

Drinking plenty of fresh, pure water is important to maintaining a healthy body and a healthy lifestyle. Water is important to maintaining optimal levels of health. Try substituting water for less healthy beverages like soda and coffee. Strive for 8 cups of water each day.

Am I able to maintain my optimal body weight?

Gaining weight without trying to is often a sign of a poor diet. Following a healthy diet, and getting plenty of regular exercise, is the only way to lose weight and keep it off.

Do I limit the amount of salt, sugar, alcohol and caffeine in my diet?

While all of these elements are fine in moderation, excessive amounts of any of these four can indicate a serious problem with your diet. It is important to limit the amount of unhealthy elements in any diet.

Variety – Your Key to a Healthy Diet

It has been said that variety is the spice of life, and that is certainly true when trying to eat a healthy diet. No one likes to eat the same thing day after day, and boredom is the enemy of a healthy diet.

Fortunately for those trying to follow a healthy diet, there is plenty of variety to be had in healthy foods. In addition to the hundreds of varieties of fruits and vegetables available at the average grocery store, there is a wide variety of beans, lentils, nuts, meat, dairy products, fish and poultry. There is no need for boredom to set in when pursuing a healthier lifestyle.'

The key to enjoying a variety of foods while eating healthy is to plan meals carefully and be sure to use the many varieties of foods that are available. Using a combination of fresh fruit, vegetables, meats and whole grains, it is possible to create a fresh, exciting and healthful meal every day of the week.

Nutritionists often stress the importance of a varied diet, both for nutritional and psychological reasons. A varied diet is essential for good health, since different types of foods contain different types of nutrients. And following a varied diet is important to your psychological well being as well, since feeling deprived of your favorite foods can lead you to give up your healthy lifestyle.

It is much better to continue eating the foods you like, but to eat them in moderation. Instead of giving up that juicy bacon, for instance, have it as an occasional treat, perhaps pairing it with an egg white omelet instead of a plateful of scrambled eggs with the yolk.

It is important for everyone to eat foods from the five major food groups each and every day. The five food groups identified by the USDA include grains, vegetables, fruits, milk and dairy and meat and beans. Each of these food groups contains specific nutrients, so it is important to eat a combination of these foods to ensure proper levels of nutrition.

Of course simply choosing foods from the five food groups is not enough. After all a meal from the five food groups could include cake, candied yams, avocados, ice cream and bacon. Although all five food groups are represented, no one would try to argue that this is a healthy day's menu. Choosing the best foods from within each group, and eating the less healthy foods in moderation, is the best way to ensure a healthy diet.

For instance, choosing healthy, lean meats is a great way to get the protein you need without consuming unnecessary fat and calories. Turkey, chicken, and fish are good sources of protein. Also, removing fat and skin from chicken is a great way to eliminate extra fat and calories.

When choosing breads and cereals, it is usually best to choose those that carry the whole grain designation. Whole grains, those that have not been overly refined, contain greater nutritional qualities and fewer sugars.

In addition, many grains and cereals are fortified with additional vitamins and minerals. While this vitamin fortification is important, it should be seen as a bonus, not as a substitute for a proper diet. Many foods are supplemented with important nutrients such as calcium (essential for strong bones and teeth) and folic acid (important in preventing birth defects).

No matter what your reason for following a healthy diet, or what your ultimate fitness goals may be, you will find that a good understanding of nutrition will form the basis of your healthy diet. Understanding how the various food groups work together to form a healthy diet will go a long way toward helping you meet your ultimate fitness goals. Whether your goal is to run a marathon, lose ten pounds or just feel better, knowledge is power, and nutritional knowledge will power your diet for the rest of your life.

A Variety of Foods for a Healthy Lifestyle

Of course simply eating foods from a variety of sources is not enough. It is also important to make smart choices within those food groups. After all, nonfat yogurt and a hot fudge sundae are both dairy products! The best choice in that situation should be obvious, but other choices are more subtle.

Fortunately, the nutritional labels which are required on all packaged foods are a big help for those pursuing a healthier diet. Not only do these labels contain information on the number of calories, fat grams, etc., but they provide detailed information on the levels of many vitamins and nutrients.

When choosing healthy foods, small changes can have a huge impact. Replacing highly processed grains for more nutritious whole grain products can also have a great impact on healthy eating. In nutritional terms, less is often more – that is less processing and less refining. Processing and refining methods can strip many vital nutrients from foods, so choosing less refined whole grain foods is important.

Cooking techniques are also very important when maximizing the health benefits of the foods you choose. After taking the time to choose the healthiest, freshest broccoli in the supermarket, it would be quite a waste to slather that cooked broccoli with cheese and butter, for instance.

It would also be a mistake to overcook that broccoli, especially by boiling it in water for a long time. That is because vegetables can lose significant amounts of nutrients through overcooking. When preparing fresh vegetables, it is best to quickly steam them in the microwave or on the stove, using as little water as possible. Use only enough water to keep the vegetables from scorching.

When cooking potatoes, it is a good idea to eat the entire potato, including the skin. Potato skins contain significant levels of nutrients, including fiber, vitamins and minerals. Cooking a baked potato in the microwave, or on the grill, is a great way to make the skin moist and delicious. In addition, these methods of cooking minimize the need for high fat butter or sour cream to flavor the potato. In place of these high fat options, why not use a dollop of plain nonfat yogurt, or some low fat cottage cheese?

Planning Healthy Meals

Planning healthy meals can be difficult and time consuming, but with some advance planning and some basic knowledge of nutrition, it is easy to create a week's worth of healthy meals that everyone in the family will love.

The key to creating healthy, delicious meals for the family is planning, planning and planning. Planning the week's meals ahead of time is the best way to create meals you can be proud of, while keeping cost and time commitment to a minimum.

Convenience devices such as slow cookers and microwaves can be a huge time saver when planning and preparing meals. There are many delicious and healthy recipes that can be started in the morning and left to cook all day in a crock pot or slow cooker. These are great choices for working families.

In addition, making the meals ahead of time on the weekend and heating them in the microwave is a great way to stretch both your food and your time. There are many microwavable healthy meals you can make at home, and single serving microwave safe containers allow every member of the family to eat on their own schedule.

When planning the meals for the week, it is a good idea to create a chart listing each day's menu and each day's schedule. Planning the quickest, easiest to prepare meals for the busiest days of the week is a smart strategy.

It is a good idea to involve the entire family in creating the week's meal plan. Get everyone's input and note everyone's favorite foods. Of course, that does not mean eating pizza every night or having ice cream for dinner. It is still important to eat healthy meals, and involving your spouse and children in healthy meal planning is a great way to pique their interest in healthy eating at an early age.

It is also a good idea to get the entire family involved in the preparation of the meals. Even children too young to cook can help out by setting out the dishes, chopping vegetables, clearing the table and washing the dishes.

Cooking large quantities of healthy food is a great way to save time. Cooking large amounts of stews, soups, pasta, chili and casseroles can be a huge time saver. Making double and even triple batches of these staple foods, and freezing the leftovers for later use, is a great way to save both time and money.

When freezing leftovers, however, it is important to label the containers carefully, using freezer tape and a permanent marker. Try to keep the oldest foods near the top to avoid having to throw away expired items.

Stocking up on meats when they are on sale is another great way to use that valuable freezer space. Stocking up on such easily frozen foods as chicken, turkey, ground beef, steaks, roasts and chops is a great way to make your food dollar stretch as far as possible while still allowing you and your family to enjoy healthy, delicious meals every day.

 Keeping a well stocked pantry is as important as keeping a well stocked freezer. Stocking the pantry with a good supply of staple items like canned vegetables, canned fruits, soup stocks, rice, and other long lasting foods will make healthy meal preparation much faster and easier.

Stocking the pantry can save you money as well as time. Grocery stores are always running sales, and these sales are a great time to stock up. Buying several cases of canned vegetables when they are on sale, for instance can save lots of money and provide the basic ingredients for many nutritious, easy to prepare meals.

Examples of great staples to stock up on include whole grain cereals, pastas, tomato sauce, baked beans, canned salmon, tuna and whole grain breads. It is easy to combine these staples into many great meals on a moment's notice.

The Notion of Moderation

The key to the success of any plan for healthy eating is to eat what you like, but to exercise moderation when it comes to the less healthy foods. Improving your level of health and fitness does not mean forgoing that piece of chocolate cake, for instance. It does mean, however, limiting yourself to one piece. A healthy diet contains all types of foods, including carbohydrates, proteins, and even fats. The key is choosing foods that provide the best combination of taste and nutrition. After all, if your diet consists of foods you hate, you will not stick with it.

The revised USDA food pyramid contains five major food groups – grains, vegetables, fruits, milk and dairy, and meat and beans. When choosing foods from these groups, it is important to eat a wide variety of foods from every food group. Doing so will not only give you a great deal of variety and keep boredom from setting in, but it will provide the best nutritional balance as well. In addition to the widely known micronutrients, such as vitamin A, vitamin D, vitamin C, etc. all foods contain a variety of other elements that are vital to proper nutrition. Though present in extremely tiny amounts, those elements are vitally important to good health. That is why a healthy, varied diet is so important.

In addition, when choosing foods from within the various food groups, some choices are naturally better and healthier than others. For instance, choosing skim or 2% milk instead of full fat whole milk is a good way to cut down on both fat and calories. And choosing poultry or lean meat is a great way to get the protein you need every day without extra fat, cholesterol and calories. Even in the world of fruits and vegetables some choices are better than others. For instance, peaches packed in heavy syrup add unnecessary sugar to the diet, while those packed in water are more nutritious.

There has been a trend lately to add vitamin fortification to food, and this can sometimes be a good way to maximize nutrition. It is important to remember, however, that proper nutrition comes from a healthy diet, not from vitamin supplements. It is fine to buy calcium fortified cereal, but the bulk of your calcium intake should still come from milk, dairy products and green leafy veggies.

Nutrition Trends and Goals

The past few years have seen a bit of a resurgence of interest in healthy living and healthy eating, and that is a good thing. We all know that most people do not eat enough fruits and vegetables, and that many people eat too much of the wrong things – like sugar, salt and fat. Reversing this trend will take some time and some effort, but starting with your own diet is a great way to improve your health and your life.

The key to changing your diet, of course, is to change it is ways that you can live with for a lifetime. The reason that most diet and lifestyle changes fail is that they are too difficult to follow once the initial excitement has worn off. The key is to make small changes that you can follow for the rest of your life.

Where you start your healthy eating plan depends in great part on your particular goals. For many people, a healthy eating program can be as simple as eating more fruits and vegetables. For others, a healthy eating plan will require a radical change in the way they shop, cook, and eat.

Since healthy eating means so many different things to different people, it is impossible to come up with a single healthy eating guide that will be right for everyone. The runner toning up for a marathon will have different nutritional needs than the factory worker who wants to lose 20 pounds.

No matter what the goal, however, it is important to eat a variety of foods, and to make smart choices when shopping, when cooking and when eating. Eating out can present special challenges, and it is important to familiarize yourself with the ingredients of the foods you order in your favorite restaurant.

Making healthy food choices means eating more of the good foods – like vegetables, fruits, whole grains, etc., and less of the bad foods, like salt, sugar and fats.

Starting by eating more high nutrition, low calorie foods is a good place to start. Luckily, the produce section of the local grocery store likely contains hundreds of different examples of such foods. Fruits and vegetables are almost always low in calories and fat, and they are generally very nutritious as well.

Since variety is so important to a healthy diet, it is a good idea to try out a sampling of different fruits and vegetables on your first healthy eating shopping trip. Start with some of the fruits and vegetables you have always wanted to try but never gotten around to. For instance, many people have never tasted asparagus, spinach or Brussels sprouts. While some love these foods and others hate them, you will never know unless you try them for yourself.

This kind of foraging is a great way to introduce yourself to foods you have never tried before. It is a great way to try new things, and you just might discover a new favorite food while you're at it.

Experimenting with cooking all these exotic fruits and vegetables is another great idea. There are a ton of healthy cooking recipes and cookbooks on the market, and a new cookbook can be a great motivator for healthy eating.

It is important to remember that making your diet healthier does not necessarily mean making a radical change. Simple changes, like trimming the excess fat off of a steak, or substituting nonfat yogurt for sour cream on your baked potato, can go a long way toward enjoying a healthier lifestyle.

As a matter of fact, in the long run the simplest and easiest to follow changes are the ones that matter most. That is because making easy changes means that you will be able to stick with them for the long run. Healthy eating is a marathon, not a sprint.

Healthy Snacks

Snacking is one of those issues that can wreck the best laid plan for healthier eating. Everyone wants a snack now and then, but the key is to make those snacks healthy and nutritious as well as delicious. There are many great snacks that can be enjoyed guilt free. For instance choosing snacks from whole grain products, fruits and vegetables, milk and dairy products, meat and nuts can be a great way to satisfy your craving without destroying your diet.

The world of grain and whole grain products contain a great many healthy snacks, including whole grain breads (wheat bread and rye bread are great choices), whole what bagels, wholesome tortilla shells, pita bread and whole grain cereals.

The all important vegetable and fruit food group contains so many ideas for healthy snacks that it would be impossible to list them all here. Some of the best, tastiest and easiest fresh fruit and vegetable snacks include baby carrots or carrot slices, bit size vegetables such as broccoli florets, radishes and green peppers, fresh vegetable and fruit juice and fruit salads.

Of course fresh fruit also makes a great snack on its own. Snacking on apples, bananas and oranges is a great way to eat healthy and still enjoy delicious snacks. Keeping a bowl of delicious fruit on the table or the coffee table is a great way to encourage the entire family to eat healthier.

The milk and dairy products food group also contains many healthy snack items, including low fat and nonfat yogurt, skim milk, low fat puddings, cheeses and even chocolate milk.

Low fat cuts of prepared meats and low fat varieties of lunch meats make great snacks as well. Sandwiches made with whole grain bread and low calorie spreads like mustard can be a great treat any time of day or night.

Canned tuna (packed in water of course), peanut butter, eggs and egg substitutes, poultry, nuts and beans are also excellent choices for healthy snacks.

When creating healthy snacks, it is important to limit the consumption of high fat foods, and foods high in salt and sodium. Instead of buying snacks in the snack aisle of the grocery store, try making your own using some of the suggestions listed above.

For added variety, try combining several different healthy snacks in unexpected ways. For instance, try spreading peanut butter on pita bread, or use it as a fun dip for apple slices. Or top a whole grain English muffin with tuna and cheese. Place it in the broiler for a few minutes and enjoy a healthy and delicious snack.

Other good ideas for quick and healthy snacks include pairing fresh fruit with nonfat plain or vanilla yogurt, adding fresh fruit slices to cereal, and using fresh fruit and fruit juices to make delicious smoothies.

To perk up bagels that are getting a little stale, try slicing them into thin pieces and arranging them on a baking sheet. Brush them with some low fat salt free butter or margarine, some garlic powder and bake them for 10-12 minutes at 350 degrees. This is a great way to make your own inexpensive and healthy bagel chips without the preservatives or extra sodium found in the store bought variety. There are of course many other types of healthy snacks, and their variety is only limited by your creativity. It is important to make a variety of healthy snacks, and keep them readily at hand.

Brown Bagging your Lunch

When enjoying a healthy lifestyle, one of the biggest challenges is making meals on the go. Brown bagging is even more difficult when children are involved, but it is still possible to create delicious, nutritious brown bag lunches that the whole family will love.

The most important part of creating healthy, delicious brown bag lunches is choosing the foods that will go into those brown bags. It is important to choose foods that are easy to put together, and to include foods that everyone in the family likes. Including everyone's favorite foods is a great way to make sure the lunches will be eaten instead of traded for Twinkies.

When creating healthy brown bag lunches for yourself and your family, try to choose at least three choices from the following list.

- At least one fruit or vegetable, either fresh, canned or frozen. Some good choices include apples, bananas, oranges or fruit salad.
- A whole grain product like bread, a tortilla shell, a bagel, pasta, rice or muffins.
- Milk or dairy products like low fat or nonfat yogurt, skim milk, cheese or a yogurt drink or shake.
- Meat, fish, poultry, eggs, peanut butter, legumes or hummus
- A healthy vegetable or fruit salad

It is a great idea to involve the whole family in the preparation of these brown bag creations. Why not have a family session where everyone creates their own healthy brown bag lunches using the ingredients you provide? Lay out all the healthy foods, selected from the above list, and let everyone choose their favorites. Involving the kids in meal planning at an early age is a great way to help them learn to make healthy food choices throughout their lives.

Packing those brown bag lunches can be exciting and fun for the whole family. For instance, why not let every member of the family choose his or her own special lunch box or bag? Other good ideas and tips for brown bag lunches include setting aside one shelf in the fridge for lunch fixings and finished lunches, and setting aside a drawer in the cupboard for packaging, such as plastic bags, plastic cutlery, and napkins.

Of course, keeping the variety in brown bag lunches is very important, both for the adults and the kids. There are some great suggestions for keeping everyone from getting bored:

- Use a variety of different breads in your sandwiches. Use a combination of wheat bread, rye bread and pumpernickel, in addition to interesting bread alternatives such as tortilla wraps, bread sticks and whole wheat crackers.
- Pack bite size vegetables, such as baby carrots, broccoli florets and pepper slices, along with a low fat dipping sauce.
- Add bit size fruit like grapes, blueberries, orange

wedges and strawberries.

- Use only 100% fruit juice in brown bag lunches. Avoid fruit drinks and blends, which often contain less than 10% real fruit.
- Pick up a variety of single serving cereal and let everyone choose their favorites.
- Buy a good selection of flavors of nonfat or low fat yogurt every week, and let everyone choose their favorite flavor every day.

One great way to enjoy a variety of healthy new foods is to form a lunch partnership with four or five other coworkers. Everyone takes turns bringing lunch for everyone. This can be a great way to enjoy healthy new foods and get some new recipes.

Understanding Fats and Carbohydrates

Fats and carbohydrates are two building blocks of a healthy diet, but many people do not understand their role in proper nutrition. While the daily intake of fats and oils should be limited, these elements are still a vital part of the diet. The key is to make smart choices when it comes to fats and oils. That means substituting saturated fats with unsaturated fats, and using healthier, lighter oils in cooking.

Let's look at the role fats and oils play in the diet. Fats are necessary for supplying energy storage to the body. In addition, fats supply essential fatty acids and act as carriers for fat soluble vitamins like vitamin A, vitamin D, vitamin E, vitamin K and the carotenoids. In addition, fats have an important role to play as building blocks for various tissues and membranes, and they also play a key role in regulating numerous bodily functions.

Dietary fat is available from a variety of plant and animal sources, and most diets do contain adequate amounts of fat. Most nutrition experts recommend keeping the intake of fat to less than 20% of calories, but studies have shown that severely limiting fat intake can be dangerous.

The type and amount of fat in the diet makes all the difference. A diet high in saturated fats, trans fats and cholesterol has been associated with a variety of ills, including heart disease, stroke and other associated diseases. In addition, many long term chronic problems, such as obesity, are associated with high levels of dietary fats.

The greatest risk of complications from excessive fat intake appears to lie with saturated fats and trans fats (fats that are solid at room temperature). One of the best ways to keep levels of saturated fat low is to limit the amount of animal fats that are consumed. These animal based fats include meats like bacon and sausage, as well as butter and ice cream. Dietary cholesterol can be limited by watching the consumption of eggs, organ meats and other foods high in cholesterol.

Food labels do make the complicated process of choosing the right fats somewhat easier. For instance, trans fats will be listed on the ingredient list of foods that contain them. In general, trans fats are found mainly in processed foods.

Some fats, such as polyunsaturated fats and monounsaturated fats, are better choices for healthy eating. Examples of these fats include canola oil and olive oil. Cooking with these lighter oils can be a big step toward a healthier diet. Polyunsaturated and monounsaturated fats are liquid at room temperature, and they have been found to have heart protecting qualities.

Many types of fish have also been found to be sources of good fat. Fish are excellent sources of omega-3 fatty acids. These omega-3's have been found to promote good health, and they may even lower cholesterol levels.

Carbohydrates are an important part of a healthy diet as well, and carbs are necessary for providing energy and many essential nutrients. Carbohydrates are found in fruits and vegetables, in grains and in milk and dairy products. It is important to choose carbohydrates carefully, however, since not all are equally healthy.

When choosing breads and cereal, for instance, try to select those made with whole grains, while avoiding the more highly refined varieties. It is also important to limit the intake of sugars, such as soda, candy and highly processed baked goods. Consuming large amounts of such high calorie, low nutrient foods, can make it very difficult to stay on a healthy diet without gaining weight.

Most Americans tend to have too much of certain elements in their diet. Sugar is one such element and salt is the other. While a basic level of sodium in the form of salt is important to proper nutrition, most people consume too much salt in their daily diet. Excess salt consumption can lead to water retention, high blood pressure and other complications.

Antioxidants the Natural Way

You may have about the importance of antioxidants in the diet, and their possible role in fighting a variety of illnesses, including some kinds of cancer, age related degeneration and heart disease.

You could also be forgiven for thinking that antioxidant vitamins are things that come in pills, powders and capsules. The marketing of antioxidant vitamin supplements, such as vitamin A, vitamin C and vitamin E, is intense and relentless. While vitamin supplements can be helpful, however, the majority of antioxidant vitamins should come from food, not from vitamin supplements.

It is important to understand how antioxidant vitamins work to protect the body from harm. Antioxidants work by combining with and neutralizing harmful elements known collectively as free radicals. Free radicals are produced naturally by the body, as a consequence of a number of natural bodily processes. Most of the time, the body is able to neutralize and eliminate these free radicals on its own.

However, stresses such as environmental pollution, a weakened immune system, UV radiation and alcohol consumption can lower the body's ability to fight these free radicals.

Excessive free radicals in the human body can cause damage to the structure and function of the various organs and systems in the body. Recent studies have implicated free radicals in a number of diseases, including cancer and heart disease. In addition, free radicals are thought to play a significant role in the aging process.

It is estimated that foods contain some 4,000 different compounds that have antioxidant qualities. Since only a small number of these compounds have been identified, and a lesser amount yet have been synthesized, it is easy to see why it is so hard for vitamin supplements to replace a healthy diet. Healthy, antioxidant containing foods like fruits, vegetables and whole grains, contain a variety of trace elements and other micronutrients in addition to the antioxidant vitamins that have been identified by science.

<u>Sources of the Major Antioxidant Vitamins:</u>

Vitamin C

Vitamin C is probably the most studied of all the antioxidant vitamins. Also known as ascorbic acid, vitamin C is a water soluble vitamin found in all bodily fluids, and it is thought to be one of body's first lines of defense against infection and disease. Since vitamin C is a water soluble vitamin, it is not stored and must be consumed in adequate quantities every day. Good dietary sources of vitamin C include citrus fruits such as oranges and grapefruits, green peppers, broccoli and other green leafy vegetables, strawberries, cabbage and potatoes.

Vitamin E

Vitamin E is a fat soluble vitamin that is stored in the liver and other tissues. Vitamin E has been studied for its effects on everything from delaying the aging process to healing a sunburn. While vitamin E is not a miracle worker, it is an important antioxidant, and it is important that the diet contain sufficient amounts of vitamin E. Good dietary sources of this important nutrient include wheat germ, nuts, seeds, whole grains, vegetable oil, fish liver oil and green leafy veggies.

Beta-carotene

Beta-carotene is the nutrient that gives flamingos their distinctive pink color (they get it from the shrimp they eat). In the human world, beta-carotene is the most widely studied of over 600 carotenoids that have thus far been discovered. The role of beta-carotene in nature is to protect the skins of dark green, yellow and orange fruits from the damaging effects of solar radiation. Scientists believe that beta-carotene plays a similar protective role in the human body. Sources of beta-carotene in the diet include such foods as carrots, squash, sweet potatoes, broccoli, tomatoes, collard greens, kale, cantaloupe, peaches and apricots.

Selenium

Selenium is one of the most important minerals in a healthy diet, and it has been studied for its ability to prevent cell damage. Scientists see this ability to protect cells from damage as possibly important in the prevention of cancer, and selenium is being studied for possible cancer preventative properties. It is important to get the selenium you need from your diet, since large doses of selenium supplements can be toxic. Fortunately, selenium is easily found in a healthy diet. Good sources of dietary selenium include fish and shellfish, red meat, whole grains, poultry and eggs, and garlic. Vegetables grown in selenium rich soils are also good sources of dietary selenium.

Healthy Eating for a Healthy Body

Healthy eating means many things to many people, and everyone has different goals for the perfect diet. The key to following a healthy diet is to find a diet you can stick with for the rest of your life. A diet should not be simply a temporary change in the way you life, eat and exercise. Rather, it should be a permanent change that you can live with day in and day out, year in and year out.

For some people, a healthy diet can be as simple as increasing the amount of fruits and vegetables in the daily diet. For others, a radical change, involving strict control of fat and cholesterol, may be required.

Of course what is needed will depend on the goal of each individual. The serious runner in search of greater conditioning will of course have different goals than the couch potato who is concerned about the possibility of heart disease.

Even though every person will different goals when it comes to healthy eating, the basic tenets of healthy eating are the same. The most important thing is to eat a good variety of foods, while eating less of the bad stuff and more of the good.

That may sound like an oversimplification, but it really is that easy. Putting that simple concept into proactive, however, is the hard part. Everyone wants to eat healthier, but there are so many temptations in today's world that healthy eating can be very difficult. The key is to make healthy choices as appealing as unhealthy ones.

One way to make healthy foods appealing is buying a wide variety of exotic fruits at the local supermarket. There are probably varieties of fruits and vegetables at your local grocery store that you never even heard of before. Why not make your next trip to the grocery store an adventure by sampling these exotic offerings?

Experimenting with new recipes is another great way to bring excitement and adventure to healthy eating. A quick perusal of your favorite low fat or healthy eating cookbook will likely present you with many fun and exciting recipes to try. Often a new cookbook, or a couple of new recipes are all it takes to spur a healthier lifestyle.

It is also important to know that eating healthier does not necessarily mean making a radical change. There are very simple things you can do, such as cutting the skin off your chicken breast, or trimming the fat from your favorite steak, that can result in significant fat reductions and health improvements.

Other examples of small changes resulting in healthier eating include:

- Replacing whole milk with skim or 2%, both in recipes and for drinking
- Snacking on sorbet or low fat frozen yogurt instead of premium ice cream
- Spraying pans with nonfat cooking spray instead of using butter or margarine
- Replacing high fat cuts of meat with leaner ones
- Eating more low fat fish and less red meat
- Using egg substitutes in recipes, meals and baking

There are probably hundreds of other such tips, and they can add up to significant health improvements, whether your goal is to get fit, lose weight or improve your level of health. No matter who you are or what your current level of fitness, eating a healthier diet and losing weight may be easier than you think.

In the end, eating a healthy diet, improving your level of fitness, and managing your consumption of fat and cholesterol boils down to common sense. Depriving yourself of your favorite foods can be counterproductive to a long term dietary change. Deprivation leads inevitably to cravings, and that can start a vicious cycle of dieting and splurging. It is best to think of healthy eating as a marathon rather than a sprint. The goal of any healthy eating program should be to make easy, lifelong changes in the way you shop, cook and eat. Only by making changes that last a lifetime will you gain the most from a diet.

Getting the Most from Fruits and Vegetables

Fruits and vegetables are among the healthiest of all foods, and the great variety of these foods at the local grocery store makes it easier than ever to enjoy great meals and snacks anytime the mood strikes you.

The latest food guidelines recommend that adults eat from five to nine servings of fruits and vegetables every day. While that may seem like a lot, it is an important goal to strive for, and a very reachable one.

A serving of a fruit or vegetable is equal to:

- 1 medium sized vegetable or fruit (such as an apple, orange or banana)
- 2 small fruits (such as kiwi fruit or plums)
- ½ cup of fresh, frozen or canned fruits or vegetables
- ½ cup of 100% fruit juice
- ¼ cup of dried fruit
- 1 cup of green salad

Eating a diet that is rich in fruits and vegetables is a great way to start a healthier lifestyle. Diets high in fruits and vegetables have been shown to reduce the risk of heart disease, diabetes, stroke and even some kinds of cancer. Diets high in fruits and vegetables are also important in maintaining a healthy weight.

Since different varieties of fruits and vegetables contain different types and levels of nutrients, it is important to each a good variety of fruits and vegetables. Eating a good combination of yellow, orange, red and green fruits and vegetables is a great way to ensure adequate levels of nutrition.

Fruits and vegetables are also an important source of fiber. One way to maximize the amount of fiber you get from fruits and vegetables is to eat the entire fruit and vegetable including the edible peel. Eating fruits and vegetables whole, instead of simply drinking fruit juice, is the best way to enjoy the fiber these foods have to offer. Orange juice may be very healthy, but it does not contain the same amount of fiber as an orange.

Getting sufficient fiber in the diet offers a great many health benefits, including aiding in digestion, lowering levels of cholesterol in the blood, reducing the risk of heart disease and stroke, and reducing the chances of some forms of cancer. In addition, fiber is thought to play an important role in controlling levels of blood sugar in diabetics. Fiber also helps dieters feel full while limiting the number of calories you consume.

Many people wonder if canned and frozen fruits and vegetables are as healthy and nutritious as the fresh varieties. The simple answer to this question is yes. Canned and frozen fruits and vegetables contain just as many vitamins and minerals as their fresh counterparts, so it is fine to replace fresh fruits and vegetables with canned and frozen varieties when fresh ones are not available.

How vegetables and fruits are prepared is just as important as how they are chosen. It is important to rinse fresh fruit and vegetables thoroughly under clean running water. This step is important in order to remove any dirt, pesticide residue or bacterial contamination. The outermost leaves of lettuce and cabbage should be removed, and the outside of root vegetables like carrots and potatoes should be removed, especially if you plan to consume the skins of those vegetables. Vegetables and fruits should be washed right before they are used in order to keep them as fresh as possible.

The best ways to cook vegetables in order to maintain their freshness are to boil, microwave or steam the veggies until they are tender and crisp. It is best to use as little water as possible when cooking vegetables. That is because overcooking can destroy some of the valuable vitamins and minerals the vegetables contain.

Tips for Eating Frozen and Prepared Meals

When it comes to eating healthy, fresher is almost always better. In some cases, however, it is impossible to cook fresh foods every night. For people on the go, frozen foods can be healthy alternatives to fresh products.

While there is no substitute for a well balanced, fresh cooked meal using plenty of fresh and healthy ingredients, healthy frozen meals can provide a quick and easy alternative for busy people and those who do not have time to cook meals from scratch.

No matter what type of diet you are following, chances are there is a frozen meal available to meet your needs. From low fat to heart healthy to vegetarian meals, there are a great many frozen dinners at the local supermarket or grocery store.

While frozen foods can be very healthy, it is important to keep a close eye out for potentially unhealthy ingredients as you shop. In particular, many frozen and prepared foods have unacceptably high levels of sodium. In addition, many frozen dinners may use preservatives to can cause allergic reaction.

When choosing from among the many brands and varieties of frozen foods on the grocery store shelf, it is important to read the nutritional labels very carefully. These government mandated nutritional labels contain a wealth of information, but it is important to understand how to read them.

Nutritional labels provide information on such important things as calorie count, number of fat grams and amount of sodium, as well as the percentages of various vitamins and minerals the food contains.

When examining those nutritional labels, it is important to pay close attention to the portion size. Even a small frozen dinner can be equal to two servings, so if you plan to eat the whole thing yourself, be sure to double the calories, sodium and fat content numbers.

When looking at the amount of fat in a frozen dinner, it is important to follow the widely accepted recommendations to keep the total amount of daily fat to less than 30% of daily calories. Luckily, the new nutritional labels mandated by the government makes this calculation a lot easier. Food manufacturers are required to list the amount of fat their foods contain as a percentage of an average daily diet, so it is easy to tell at a glance if a particular frozen food is a healthy, low fat choice.

In addition to keeping total fat to less than 30% of total calories, it is important to keep saturated fat levels to less than 10% of daily calories. For sodium levels, it is important to limit the amount of sodium to less than 200 milligrams for every 100 calories of food.

In addition, most experts recommend keeping your daily sodium intake to less than 2400 milligrams per day. It is important to read the labels on all frozen foods, even if they are labeled as healthy. While claiming the healthy label obligates food manufacturers to follow certain guidelines, it is still important to review the labels in order to choose the healthiest choices.

When choosing the healthiest meals from among the hundreds of varieties at the average supermarket or grocery store, it is a good idea to choose those that contain at least a half cup of vegetables, fruits or beans. Doing so will help you ensure that the meal you choose is healthy and nutritious.

Finally, since you are in the grocery store already, why not make a stop at the salad bar for a healthy addition to your frozen entrée. Many large grocery store chains have installed wonderful salad bars stocked full of fruits, vegetables and low fat dressings

Stocking a Fridge with Health Foods

In many ways the refrigerator is the cornerstone of any healthy eating plan. How you stock that fridge can make a huge difference in the success or failure of any healthy eating plan. From what foods it contains, to where they are stored, the refrigerator can be vitally important to healthy eating.

The first step should be to take stock of just what the refrigerator contains. The bachelors among us may already be familiar with this process, but taking stock of the fridge means more than just throwing away those foods that have begun to turn green or grow hair.

Taking stock of the contents of the fridge should mean a monthly review of everything it contains. During this review, separate the healthier foods from the others. It is important to make sure that you have more low fat, high fiber and low sugar foods than high fat low fiber and high sugar ones. If the ratio is off, try to shop for healthier foods.

Another great trick for keeping a healthy refrigerator is to hide the less healthy foods. Try hiding the desserts and other such foods in the crisper, where they will be out of sight and not constantly tempting you. Since fresh fruits and vegetables tend to dry out if they are not used right away, store them in plain sight to increase their likelihood of being eaten. Hiding cakes in the produce drawers, and prominently displaying the fruits and vegetables, is a smart way to keep a healthy fridge.

Another tip is to organize the refrigerator into different sections, and to segregate those sections into sometimes foods (unhealthy choices) and everyday foods (healthy choices). Try to place the healthier foods in the front of the refrigerator, while relegating the unhealthier choices to the back.

Substitution is another great strategy for creating a healthy fridge and a healthy lifestyle. There are low fat and nonfat versions of literally hundreds of different foods. Try substituting skim or 1% milk for whole milk, soft margarines for fattier butter, and low fat sour cream for the full fat varieties. Try replacing fattier meats with leaner ones, or with chicken and fish. Even a simple change, like substituting a soft margarine for butter, can result in significant savings of saturated fat.

Try storing healthy foods with attractive, delicious toppings to make them more interesting and appealing to young children. Try storing a container of berries or sweet granola next to the low fat yogurt, or a bottle of chocolate syrup with the 1% milk.

Making Smart Food Choices with Practical Foods

Everyone who is trying to follow a healthy eating lifestyle understands the need to buy quality, healthy and practical foods. Practical foods are those foods that are not only healthy but whose benefits extend beyond their mere nutritional value. Such foods are easy to use, and useful in a number of different recipes. Healthy, practical foods, when used on a regular basis, form a great part of a healthy diet, and may even lower the risk of heart disease, cancer and other common illnesses.

One great practical food is the humble tomato. It may not look much like an orange, but the tomato is actually a citrus fruit as well. As such, tomatoes are rich in vitamin C and other antioxidants. In addition, tomatoes are a rich source of lycopene, which has shown promise in preventing certain kinds of cancer.

In addition, tomatoes are easy to use, versatile, and inexpensive. In addition to fresh, in season tomatoes, which are delicious as well as nutritious, tomatoes are available in canned and frozen varieties as well. Tomatoes can be used in so many different ways, and in so many different recipes, that it is always a good idea to have a supply of them on hand in the pantry or the fridge.

Pastas, especially the whole wheat varieties of pastas, are another great example of functional foods. Pastas can also be used in a variety of ways, from simple tomato based sauces to elaborate creations using shrimp, tuna and other seafood.

Of course, pasta dishes can be healthy or unhealthy, depending on how they are topped. Toppings such as Alfredo sauce or rich cream sauces, should be avoided when trying to follow a healthy diet. As with all foods, such heavy sauces are fine in moderation, but they should not form the bulk of your diet.

Luckily, there are lower fat alternatives to many high fat pasta sauces, and these low fat alternatives should be used whenever possible. Substituting lower fat alternatives for fatty, unhealthy foods is an important skill when it comes to creating a healthy diet.

Whole grain breads, flours and grains are also good examples of healthy, practical foods. Stocking up on these staples when they are on sale will help ensure that you have everything you need to create the most healthy recipes possible for yourself and your family.

Whole grain products should be substituted for more highly refined breads and cereals whenever possible, since whole grain breads, cereals and grains retain more of their important nutrients than do more highly refined foods.

Starting a healthy eating program using practical foods is easy. Start by taking a personal inventory of your current diet, including where it is good and where it can use some improvement. Learn to assess the personal health risks created by your current diet (your family physician can be of particular help here). A physician or dietitian can be a big help in putting together a list of healthy, easy to use, practical foods you can use to change your diet for the better.

It is also a good idea to use your interest in healthy eating to create and use exciting new recipes. There are a great many healthy eating recipes available, both on the internet and in cookbooks. Seek out some of these recipes and try using your favorite healthy staples to create some wonderful dishes.

For some ideas on how to use practical foods morning, noon and night, try some of the ideas listed on the following pages:

Breakfast:

- Include some healthy staples, and some healthy fruits in your breakfast. For instance, pair healthy oatmeal with blueberries, or whole wheat or wheat bran cereal with strawberries or bananas.
- Try mixing a healthy cereal like All Bran into your nonfat or low fat yogurt. It will perk up your plain yogurt and give it a great crunch.
- Fresh fruit is also a great addition to yogurt. Try buying plain, nonfat yogurt and mixing in your own raspberries, blueberries and strawberries. You will save money and enjoy a healthy breakfast.
- Instead of high fat butter, spread your toast with apple butter or soy nut butter instead. Always try to use whole grain varieties of bread like wheat or rye.
- Drink a glass of 100% fruit juice with breakfast every day. Orange juice, grape juice, apple juice and grapefruit juice are all great choices.
- Blend 1% milk or soy milk with fresh pineapple for a healthy, delicious breakfast smoothie. These smoothies are great for people on the go.

Lunch and dinner ideas:

- Make a great tuna salad with grated carrots, green peppers, red peppers, garlic and onion.
- Make a dish of fresh whole grain pasta and top it will homemade tomato sauce and fresh home grown herbs.
- Use healthy foods like onions and leeks, along with tomatoes, as a great side dish.
- Grill healthy fish and serve with a healthy side salad.
- Try some low fat soups like spinach and broccoli soup.
- Make a great vegetable stir fry with olive oil.

Healthy snacks

- A piece of fresh fruit, like an apple, orange or banana, always makes a great snack. Keep a bowl of fruit on your kitchen counter for easy access.
- Try mixing nuts and dried fruit for a great homemade trail mix. Hikers and non hikers alike will enjoy this healthy snack.
- Treat yourself to a great glass of orange, tomato or cranberry juice before you leave the house in the morning.
- Keep a supply of broccoli florets, baby carrots and other bite size vegetables, and some healthy dip.

Buying Healthy Foods

The local grocery store is a great place to find healthy, nutritious foods. Unfortunately, it is also a place to find less healthy foods and many junk foods. Learning how to follow a healthy lifestyle means learning how to shop for the healthiest foods, and learning how to avoid temptation.

Learning to read labels is an important skill for any healthy shopper. The information on nutritional labels is very valuable, providing complete information on the percentage of many vitamins and minerals a particular food contains. In addition, nutritional information labels provide valuable information on things like the amount of calories, number of fat grams, percentage of total fat and amount of fiber each food contains. It is important to choose those foods that have the best nutritional qualities as you roam the local grocery store.

There are some important guidelines to follow to make sure that every trip to the grocery store will be a healthy experience. After all, you cannot have a healthy refrigerator or a healthy dinner table without first stocking your kitchen pantry with the healthiest foods available.

One of the best pieces of advice is probably something you have heard a million times, and that is to never go grocery shopping when you are hungry. Even if it means stopping for a quick snack on your way, it is important to not enter the supermarket while you are hungry. Hungry shoppers make bad choices, and those unhealthy choices will be around long after your hunger has abated.

Another good trick is to hit the produce section of your grocery store first. Fill up your food basket with healthy, nutritious fruits and vegetables. This way it will leave less room for all those less healthy foods when you get to them.

It is also important to always make a detailed shopping list before hitting the grocery store. A well thought out grocery list keeps you from overspending, and also helps keep you from succumbing to the temptation of less healthy junk foods. To keep a detailed list of what you need on your next shopping list, try keeping a notepad by the fridge or on the dining room table. Write down each item as you think of it, and come shopping day, you will have a complete list of everything you need to buy.

As you shop around the grocery store, it is a good idea to take advantage of the many low fat foods that fill grocery store shelves. There are low at varieties of many foods, including milk and dairy products, meats and cheeses, even cakes and pies. Most of these products contain all the taste of the full fat products, without all the fat.

When shopping for low fat foods, however, be on the lookout for extra sugar content. This is not so much a concern with milk and dairy products, but it is sometimes a concern with low fat baked goods. Some manufacturers pack their low fat baked goods with extra sugar, so it pays to be a smart label reader.

As long as you watch sugar content, however, low fat desserts and sweets are excellent choices. When grocery shopping, try to choose naturally lower fat alternatives, such as angel food cake, fig bars and vanilla wafers. Buying smaller portion sizes is another smart strategy for enjoying sweets while limiting fat and calories. Also, people tend to eat fewer candies and sweets when they are individually wrapped. The process of removing the wrapping and looking at the spare wrappers usually stops people from overeating them. If you buy bulk candy or cookies that are not wrapped there is a good chance you will eat more of them than if they were individually wrapped.

Another smart strategy is to choose whole grain breads and cereals whenever possible. Whole grains contain more fiber and other nutrients than do more processed foods, so buying whole grains makes a lot of sense.

When shopping for the healthiest cereals in the grocery store, it is helpful to understand how the cereal aisle of the typical grocery store is arranged. Shelf space at a grocery store is in high demand and short supply, and cereal manufacturers take advantages of this fact in their store shelf marketing. In general, the less healthy, sugar laden cereals are arranged at kid height, while the more adult, healthier products are on the top shelves. Choosing the healthier cereals from the top shelves is a good strategy, but it is still important to read the labels to make sure you are getting what you think you are.

Eat a Variety of Veggies

The new food guidelines issued by the United States government recommend that all Americans eat between five and nine servings of fruits and vegetables each and every day. When you first hear that number, it may seem like a lot, but it is actually much easier than you think to fit that many servings of fruits and vegetables into your daily diet. For one thing, the shelves of the grocery stores are fairly bursting with fresh fruits and vegetables. In addition, vegetables and fruits are some of the least expensive, most nutrient rich, foods in the supermarket. With all these fruits and vegetables to choose from, it is very easy to make these nutritious, delicious foods part of your daily meals and snacks.

One great way to get the nutrients you need from fruits and vegetables every day is to take full advantage of the variety of these foods available. Eating the same thing every day quickly becomes boring, so why not pick a variety of fruits and vegetables, in spice things up?

When shopping for fruits and vegetables, it is important to choose a variety of different colors. This is for more than purely artistic reasons. Different color fruits and vegetables generally have different types of nutrients, and choosing a variety of colors will help ensure you get all the vitamins and minerals you need each and every day.

Finding new recipes is another great way to ensure you get those five to nine servings of fruits and vegetables every day.

Everyone likes to try out new recipes, and a new recipe may provide you with the motivation to eat your fruits and veggies.

New recipes can also provide you the important opportunity to try out some fruits and vegetables you have never tried before. For instance, everyone has eaten oranges, but have you tried kiwi fruit or mangoes? How about spinach or kale? Trying new things is a great way to find new favorites while getting the best nutrition available.

Many people mistakenly think that they do not need to eat five to nine servings of fruits and vegetables every day if they just take a vitamin supplement. Actually, nothing could be further from the truth. That is because fruits and vegetables contain far more than the micronutrients identified by science and synthesized in vitamin pills. While these micronutrients, such as vitamin C, vitamin A and vitamin E are important to good health, so too are the hundreds of elements that have yet to be identified, but that are contained in healthy foods like fruits and vegetables. These elements are not available in any pill, they must be ingested through a healthy, balanced diet that contains plenty of fruits and vegetables.

In addition, fruits and vegetables are much less costly than vitamin pills. Fruits and vegetables are very inexpensive, especially when purchased in season and grown locally. In the long run, getting the nutrition you need from the food you eat is much less expensive, and much better for you, than popping those vitamin pills every day.

The Benefits of Citrus Fruits

There are few single food groups with as much to recommend them, and as many health benefits, as citrus fruits. Citrus fruits are packed full of a number of important vitamins and minerals, as well as fiber. In addition, citrus fruits are delicious, abundant, and usually quiet inexpensive.

Citrus fruits abound in most modern grocery stores, even in the winter months. Thanks to modern distribution networks, citrus fruits grown around the world are easily accessible in the supermarkets of this country.

Of course many people prefer locally grown citrus fruits, but when they are not available, shipped citrus is a good substitute. There is a growing season for each kind of citrus in various parts of the country, so it pays to familiarize yourself with those seasons in order to take advantage of the freshest locally grown tomatoes, oranges, grapefruits and more.

Citrus fruits are perfect anytime of the day, from a grapefruit in the morning to an orange at lunchtime to a dinner salad piled high with locally grown tomatoes.

Citrus fruits contain so many important vitamins and minerals that it would be impossible to list them all. Citrus fruits are a good example of why fresh fruits and vegetables are a better source of complete nutrition than vitamin supplements. While some of the important vitamins and nutrients contained in citrus fruits have been identified and synthesized, others, particularly the many trace minerals and other micronutrients, have not. Important nutrients in citrus fruits include:

Vitamin C

Vitamin C is the first thing that comes to mind when most people think of citrus fruits, and it is true that most citrus fruits are simply loaded with this important vitamin. Vitamin C is perhaps the most studied of all vitamins, and it has shown promise in shortening the duration of colds, helping wounds heal faster, and protecting the body from the damaging effects of free radicals.

Vitamin C is essential for healthy skin and gums, and since vitamin C is a water soluble vitamin, sufficient quantities must be consumed every day. Unlike fat soluble vitamins, vitamin C is not stored in the body. That is why eating at least a few servings a day of citrus fruits and other vitamin C rich foods is so important. Luckily, getting the recommended daily amount of vitamin C is not difficult, since a single orange contains 150% of the recommended daily intake of vitamin C.

Fiber

Fiber content is often overlooked as a benefit of citrus fruits. After all, most people picture cereals and grains when they think of fiber. Even so, citrus fruits are a good source of dietary fiber, including the all important soluble fiber. Fiber plays a vital role in digestion, and studies have indicated it may help to reduce levels of cholesterol in the blood and even reduce the risk of some kinds of cancer.

Folate (folic acid)

Folate, or folic acid as it is also known, plays a vital role in early pregnancy, so all women of child bearing age are encouraged to consume adequate amounts of this important nutrient. That is because one of the most critical times in a pregnancy takes place before the woman knows she is pregnant. In addition to its importance in preventing many neural tube birth defects, folic acid also aids in the production of mature red blood cells and helps to prevent anemia. Citrus fruits are an excellent source of folic acid.

Potassium

Oranges are particularly high in potassium, as are non citrus fruits like bananas. Potassium is vital to maintaining a proper fluid balance in the body, and for transmitting signals between nerve cells. Potassium levels can be affected by excess caffeine consumption and by dehydration, so it is important to consume adequate levels of potassium every day.

With all these things going for them, it is easy to see why citrus fruits are so important to the diet. No matter what your ultimate fitness goal, a diet rich in citrus fruits will help to get you off to the right start. And with the many varieties of citrus fruits to choose from, it is easy to spice things up and bring variety to your healthy eating plan.

Healthy Eating Without the Meat

As concerns about healthy eating have grown, so too has the interest in vegetarianism and veganism. Many nutrition experts recommend "eating low on the food chain". In plain language this means eating more grains, vegetables and fruits, and fewer meats, cheeses and other animal based products.

There are of course various levels of vegetarianism, and each type has its own unique health benefits and some health challenges as well. Of course vegetarians, like meat eaters, must still make healthy food choices. Simply eating French fries while avoiding a hamburger will not make you a healthy vegetarian.

Some people who consider themselves vegetarians still eat poultry and seafood, while others avoid all animal flesh, even fish and chicken. Most vegetarians still eat milk, dairy products and eggs. In nutritional circles these people are referred to as lacto-ovo vegetarians.

Vegans, on the other hand, avoid all animal products, including eggs, milk and dairy products, and even fabrics like silk, leather and wool. It is vegans who face the largest challenges and risks when trying to follow a healthy diet. Most vegetarian diets provide more than enough nutrition, as long as smart dietary choices are made.

The key to eating a healthy vegetarian diet is much the same as eating a healthy diet that includes meat. It all boils down to making smart food choices, understanding nutritional labels, and cooking your vegetables to maximize their nutritional value.

Choosing the foods that make up the bulk of a vegetarian diet is very important. For most vegetarians, vegetables, grains, lentils and soy products will make up the bulk of their diet, and these staples are included in many vegetarian recipes.

When cooking with soy, however, it is important to remember that tofu is relatively high in fat. The fat content of tofu dishes is often comparable to that of dishes that are made with lean cuts of meat. Those vegetarians following a low fat diet may want to limit the amount of tofu based products they eat.

The same caution applies to the nuts and seeds that can make up a large part of a vegetarian diet. Nuts and seeds are excellent sources of dietary protein, but they can be high in fat as well.

Many newly minted vegetarians worry that they will not be able to get enough protein and iron without eating meat, but for most vegetarians this is not a problem. Most diets today actually contain too much protein, and there are many non animal derived sources of protein for vegetarians to enjoy.

Proper cooking techniques are of course very important to any healthy diet. Avoiding high fat cooking methods is important, as is avoiding the use of high fat creams, butters and sauces. A vegetable stir fry cooked in healthy olive oil can be a great addition to any vegetarian menu. And a great fruit salad is both easy to make and delicious as a snack or a meal.

The only real area of concern when it comes to vegetarianism and health is the B-complex vitamins, particularly vitamin B12. Vitamin B12 is almost exclusively derived from animal based sources, so vegans, who avoid all animal products, should take a high quality vitamin B12 or B-complex vitamin supplement. It is also important for vegans to discuss their diet and lifestyle with their family physicians. As vegetarianism and veganism becomes more widespread, the amount of information on the nutritional needs of these two groups continues to grow.

Calcium is also a concern for vegans, since the primary sources of dietary calcium are milk and other dairy products. Again, calcium fortified foods such as some soy milk and certain cereals are important to maintaining a healthy vegan diet. The same is true of vitamin D, another primarily animal based nutrient.

The bottom line is that vegetarians can enjoy a very healthy lifestyle. Making vegetables, fruits, whole grains and beans the centerpiece of the diet is a smart move for many people, and a good low fat vegetarian diet can be a great way to enjoy a healthy lifestyle. However, it is important for vegetarians to plan their eating to make sure they get proper nutrients.

The Different Types of Fiber

When it comes to eating healthy and enjoying a healthier lifestyle, it is hard to overstate the importance of fiber in the diet. Even though fiber is most associated with grains, rice and breads, it is important to remember that fruits and vegetables also contain significant amounts of dietary fiber. In fact, the need for fiber is just one more reason to eat your fruits and vegetables every day.

In order to understand why dietary fiber is so important, it is a good idea to know what fiber is and what role it plays in digestion. Simply put, dietary fiber is the portion of food that the human body cannot digest. Fiber is found in foods of plant origin only; there is no fiber in meat and dairy products. Fiber plays an important role in the digestion of food, and in the elimination of waste products as they travel through the body.

Good sources of dietary fiber include grains, cereals, legumes, lentils, nuts, seeds, fruits and vegetables. As we said before, meats and dairy products do not contain any dietary fiber, so it is important to eat some plant based foods ever day to get the fiber you need.

Soluble vs. insoluble fiber

Not all fiber is the same, and fiber comes in two forms – soluble and insoluble. All plant materials contain both types of fiber, but some sources contain more of one than the other.

Eating a variety of foods rich in fiber every day will ensure you get adequate levels of both soluble and insoluble fiber.

Insoluble fiber is important in keeping people regular, and it has shown promise as well in the prevention of some types of colon and rectal cancers. Insoluble fiber is mainly found in wheat brain, some types of vegetables and in whole grain products. Some vegetables rich in insoluble fiber include carrots, peas and broccoli. The skins of fruits are also rich in insoluble fiber.

Soluble fiber, on the other hand, has shown promise in reducing levels of cholesterol in the blood, and at reducing the rate at which glucose enters the bloodstream. Soluble fiber is abundant in dried peas, lentils, beans, barley, oat bran, and in many fruits and vegetables.

How much fiber is enough?

Many people are unsure just how much dietary fiber they need every day, but most dietitians recommend that women consume between 21 and 25 grams of dietary fiber per day. For men, the recommendation is 30 to 38 grams of fiber each day.

Of course, that is easier said than done, and it is important to know which foods are high in fiber in order to boost your daily fiber consumption. In the case of packaged foods like breads and crackers, the fiber content will be listed as part of the nutritional label. In the case of fruits and vegetables, there are charts which show the fiber content of an average size piece. Some grocery stores post this information, and it is also widely available on the internet.

When increasing dietary fiber, it is best to make the increase gradual. A sudden jump in dietary fiber can lead to bloating, gas and abdominal discomfort. In addition, it is important to drink plenty of fluids, especially water, in order for fiber to have the best effect. When choosing breads and cereals, it is best to go with healthier whole grains. In general, the less processing, the healthier the foods.

Eating the skins of fruits and vegetables is a great way to increase dietary fiber. Many people like to make fruit shakes and smoothies that use the skins of their favorite fruits. This makes a delicious and nutritious way to increase fiber consumption. In addition, keeping a variety of fiber rich foods, such as apples, nuts, seeds and bran muffins, around for snacks is a great idea.

And finally, eating a wide variety of foods will ensure that you get plenty of fiber, as well as the vitamins, minerals, trace elements and other micronutrients that make a balanced diet so important.

Healthy Eating on a Budget

For many people, a limited food budget can be a real roadblock to healthy eating. It is an unfortunate fact of life that some of the lowest priced foods, from fast food value menus to cheap potato chips, are also some of the least healthy. It is possible, however, to create excellent tasting, nutritious meals, even on a tight budget.

The key to planning and creating healthy meals on a limited budget is good forward planning and solid nutritional knowledge.

Step 1 – The shopping list

Anyone who has visited a supermarket lately knows how dangerous it is to enter the store without a shopping list in hand. Shopping without a sense of what you need – and don't need – opens you up to all manner of temptation, and most of those tempting foods are not nutritious.

In addition, picking up all those extra items can easily blow your food budget and leave you without the funds to plan those healthy, nutritious meals. A good trick is to keep a note pad near the table or refrigerator. Having the notepad within easy reach makes it easy to keep track of the foods you need to stock up on.

Step 2 – Watch for sales

Most major food store chains publish weekly sales ads, usually as inserts in the local newspaper. Keeping track of these sales, and taking advantage of the low prices to stock up, is a great way to gather a cupboard full of healthy food. Once the pantry is full of fruits, vegetables and other healthy fare, it will be much easier to create healthy recipes the entire family will love. In addition, locally grown, in season fruits and vegetables are usually more of a bargain than out of season or shipped fruits and vegetables.

Step 3 – Stock up on staples

Essential staple foods, such as flour, rice, and pasta are frequently put on sale as loss leaders at major groceries. Stocking up on these essentials when prices are low is a great way to stretch any food budget.

Step 4 – Never shop when you are hungry

The old advice to never shop when you are hungry is definitely true. Shopping when you are hungry is a sure way to give into temptation, bust the food budget, and stock up on bad foods.

Step 5 – Become a label guru

Nutritional labels contain a wealth of information, but it is up to each shopper to read those labels and understand what they mean. Nutritional labels contain complete information on not just calories and fats, but the amounts of various essential vitamins and minerals as well. It is important to know how to read labels in order to get the best nutritional bang for your food bucks.

Step 6 – Pay close attention to package sizes

Just because two cans look alike it does not mean they are. Packaging can be deceptive, so get in the habit of comparing weights when shopping for canned fruits, vegetables and other items. Also take advantage of the lower prices available on store brand and generic products.

Step 7 – Use coupons, but do it wisely

Manufacturers coupons can be a great deal when used on products you already buy. Buying something simply because you have a coupon, however, is typically not a good idea.

Step 8 – Replace meat with beans and other substitutes

Eating less meat and more beans and lentils is a good way to save money on your food budget while still getting the protein you and your family need. Try experimenting with some vegetarian recipes for interesting ways to use these alternatives.

In addition to the tips listed above, there are several ways that smart shoppers keep their food budgets at a minimum while preparing delicious, nutritious meals for their family every day. One trick is to keep the refrigerator and the pantry well stocked with staple foods. Keeping a good supply of staples on hand will avoid unnecessary trips to the store and also avoid the need to buy such products when they are not on sale. When staples such as bread, flour, peanut butter, canned vegetables, etc. are on sale, be sure to stock up.

Healthy Eating and Dining Out

One of the biggest challenges facing those trying to follow a healthy diet is the local restaurant. Eating out presents special challenges, such as not knowing how the food was prepared, how much fat it contains, and whether or not the healthiest ingredients were used.

Many restaurant chains, and even some fast food restaurants, have recognized the demand for healthier menu choices, and they are working hard to satisfy that demand. All too often, however, the healthy choices on a restaurant menu are limited and unappealing. It is important, therefore to pay close attention to the menu and make the healthiest choices possible.

One of the most important thing diners can do to eat healthy at restaurants is to be proactive. Diners should not be afraid to ask how a dish is prepared, or what ingredients are used in its preparation. If the server does not know, ask him or her to check with the chef. A good chef will be happy to answer such questions, and to make modifications in the recipe if needed. In addition, most restaurants will happily accommodate special needs, such as low fat or low sodium dishes.

Some of our favorite tips for healthy eating in restaurants include:

- One good rule of thumb to use when dining out is to order entrees that are grilled, baked or broiled. Deep fried dishes are best avoided. If you are unsure how a dish is prepared, don't be afraid to ask.
- Portion size is just as important at the restaurant as they are at home. That means ordering the petit fillet instead of the full size steak, requesting half size portions of French fries, and maybe even forgoing that tempting dessert. Choosing leaner cuts of meat or fish is also a good way to eat healthier.
- When choosing side dishes, ask if steamed vegetables are available. Steamed veggies are an excellent, low fat, low calorie choice for many diners. Vegetables that are fried, au gratin, or prepared in cream or butter sauces are best avoided.
- When ordering salad, ask if fat free choices are available. Most restaurants have several fat free or low fat varieties of salad dressing available. If no low fat option exists, request the dressing on the side so that you can control the amount that is used.
- When ordering soup, choose broth based soups, and avoid bisques or rich soups like cream of crab or cream of broccoli. A simple vegetable soup is a delicious and low fat alternative.
- Replace high fat, high calorie French fries with healthier alternatives such as fresh fruit or an unbuttered baked potato. Most restaurants will be happy to accommodate such special requests.
- In Italian restaurants, stick with the tomato based

sauces and avoid cream or heavy Alfredo sauces. A simple pesto sauce without meat is a good choice for most pasta dishes.

- When dining at oriental restaurants, go with the steamed rice and stir fried vegetable entrees. Avoid the heavy sauces and request that your meal be prepared with less oil. In addition, try to choose dishes that feature less meat and more fresh vegetables.
- Choose a light dessert of fresh fruit or sorbet. When ordering traditional desserts, order one and share it.
- Avoid "super-sizing" a meal, and choose heather options such as apple slices over French fries.

Cooking Tips

When it comes to healthy eating, sometimes how you cook is just as important as what you eat. There are definitely healthy, and less healthy, ways to prepare the healthy foods you buy.

When it comes to cooking vegetables, it is always best to use as little water as possible. That is because over cooking, especially when boiling, can destroy some of the important nutrients that make vegetables so important.

The best way to cook most vegetables is in the microwave, preferably in a special microwave vegetable steamer. Vegetables can also be lightly cooked in a microwave safe bowl, using as little water as possible.

Vegetables can be cooked on the stove top as well, but it is important to use as little water as possible when boiling vegetables. Vegetables like broccoli and Brussels sprouts are particularly susceptible to losing important nutrients.

Microwave ovens are also great for making other vegetables, especially baked potatoes. Baked potatoes get great in the microwave, with the skins getting nice and crispy and the flesh being very tender. Of course this means that less high fat toppings may be needed, so the microwave is a great way to make nutritious and delicious baked potatoes.

Grilling is another great way to make healthy, delicious meals. Grilling meats is a great, low fat way to prepare meats, and it is a great way to make vegetables and fruits as well. Vegetable kebobs are great on the grill, whether combined with lean cuts of meat or made into a meal of their own.

Your oven's broiler is another great way to create low fat meals. Broiling is a great way to prepare all kinds of meats and seafood, and broiling is a low fat cooking method as well. Broiling fish is a great, fast and easy way to prepare this staple of a healthy low fat diet, while broiling steaks and chops keep fat at a minimum while keeping taste at its highest.

The handy kitchen blender is another great way to create delicious snacks using healthy fruits and vegetables. Blenders are great for making fruit smoothies, and most recipes call for little more than crushed ice, fruit juice and fresh fruit.

Some great, high nutrition, low fat, low calorie meals require no preparation at all. For instance, it is possible to make a wonderful, and easy, fruit salad with just a can of mandarin oranges, an apple, some strawberries and a banana. Simply open the can of mandarin oranges, empty it into a bowl, along with the juice it is packed in. Then add banana slices, apples slices and strawberries. For extra color and taste, add some blueberries, raspberries or raisins. The total prep time for this great creation is all of five minutes.

Fruit skewers are another creative, healthy and easy meal or snack. Simply take shish kebob skewers and stack them full of melon slices, strawberries, red grapes, white grapes and chunks of pineapple. Plain nonfat yogurt makes an excellent and low fat dip.

In addition to the above ideas, making your own homemade salsa is a great way to create a low fat alternative to sour cream and other high fat dips. Salsa can be made using healthy ingredients like tomatoes, mangoes, avocados, onions, cilantro and lime juice.

In addition, perking up a plain salad is a great way to add even more fruits and vegetables to an already healthy diet. For example, use broccoli florets, carrot slices, slices of cucumber, green peppers, red peppers, and bean sprouts to add color, zest and flavor to any salad.

Cucumbers, green peppers, broccoli and carrots are also great additions to pasta salads and potato salads. Adding extra crunch and color is a great way to add zest to any meal or snack.

Even a plain green salad of lettuce and tomatoes can be enhanced through the use of colorful fruits and vegetables. Adding vegetables like carrots, bean sprouts, and spinach leaves, and fruits like mandarin oranges, apple slices, nectarine slices, grapes, apple slices, pineapples and raisins, adds both beauty and taste to any salad.

Of course salad dressing is always an important subject for those trying to follow a healthy lifestyle. High fat dressing can sabotage even the healthiest salad, but there are many excellent, low fat and healthy choices when it comes to topping a salad. Using flavored vinegars, herbs and fruit juices are novel approaches to salad dressing, in addition to the many nonfat and low fat versions of commercial salad dressing.

The Benefits of Fish

It is hard to beat fish and seafood for high protein and low fat. Fish has been shown in study after study to have a positive impact on health, and to lower the risk of heart disease and other diseases. In addition, fish is delicious and easy to prepare.

Many nutrition experts recommend eating fish at least once or twice every week. The most nutritious varieties of fish, and those that contain the greatest amounts of heart protecting omega-3 fatty acids, tend to be those that live in cold ocean waters. These varieties of fish include salmon and sardines.

As a matter of fact, fish is one of the best sources of protein there is. Everyone needs protein for building muscles and repairing damaged body tissues. In addition, protein plays a vital role in the growth of nails and hair, in hormone production and in many other vital bodily processes.

In addition to fish, many other animal based products, such as meat, eggs, poultry and dairy products, contain significant amounts of protein. Plant based sources of protein exist as well, in nuts, beans and lentils, among others.

The key to getting sufficient protein in the diet is to balance the healthy effects of protein on the diet against the large amounts of fat and cholesterol that protein rich foods often contain. The combination of high protein and low fat is one of the things that makes a diet rich in fish so appealing.

With the exception of salmon, almost all commonly eaten varieties of fish are very low in fat, and even salmon contains lower levels of fat than many varieties of meats. In addition, fish is low in saturated fat, the type of fat that is most associated with heart disease and clogged arteries.

Fish is low in unsaturated fat because of the nature of where and how they live. Instead of storing energy in the form of saturated fat as land animals do, fish store their fat in the form of polyunsaturated oils. That adaptation allows their bodies to function normally in the cool oceans and streams where they swim. It also makes them a great choice for anyone seeking to cut levels of saturated fat in the diet.

For all these reasons, fish remains an important part of any low fat, heart healthy lifestyle. Substituting high fat, greasy foods like hamburgers and ribs is a great way to make a change for healthy living.

One note about fish and pollution, however. It is true that many fish caught in polluted waters contain high levels of mercury. While most commercially caught and grown fish is low in mercury, it is important for fisherman to limit their consumption of locally caught fish. Pregnant women are also advised to limit their intake of fish, due to the potential harm to the baby.

Conclusion to the Healthy Eating Power Guide

Every person can experience the health benefits from a proper diet, and the payout of investing in your nutrition can be huge. With a good diet, you can lose weight, help fight off disease, avoid medical complications, improve physical ability and have more energy for day to day activities. Children, adults, senior citizens and everyone in between can find use for these benefits.

The tips and strategies in this guide were designed to point you in the right direction of proper nutrition, but it is up to you to reach your health goals. Some people may need extra help from a nutritionist to make the right food choices, and you may need extra motivation from family members, friends and support groups. Good health is not something that can be attained over night, but with enough dedication and drive you can see the benefits.

Made in the USA
Middletown, DE
27 February 2022

61883251R00076